Discover your Past Lives
a Journey of Self-Knowledge
Isis Estrada

Holos Arts Project

Discover your Past Lives

a Journey of Self-Knowledge

Isis Estrada

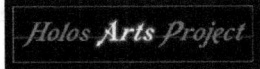

Publisher: Holos Arts Project

The purpose of this book is to present an alternative therapeutic method, which in no way should replace a medical treatment or prescribed medicine. The topics covered here are an auxiliary to any type of medical therapy and are presented as a complementary option.

About the Author:

The therapist Isis Estrada is a master in psychology and doctor in metaphysics; graduated from the University of Minnesota USA and the Antonio de Nebrija University in Spain. For several decades she has been a professor at various universities in her native Mexico; she is also the author of several books related to alternative therapies and mysticism, which have been published in Spanish and English. She is currently the general director of the Center for Alternative Therapies "Mystic Path" in Mexico City. She is also a member and authorized course provider for "The International Guild of Complementary Therapists", London, England (IGCT).

About the Publisher:

Holos Arts Project is a group dedicated to the formation, creation and diffusion of art in its different manifestations. Holos Arts Project produces books, music, photography and podcasts on topics related to art, spirituality and psychology. It is directed by Isis Estrada and Carlos Robles Cruz.

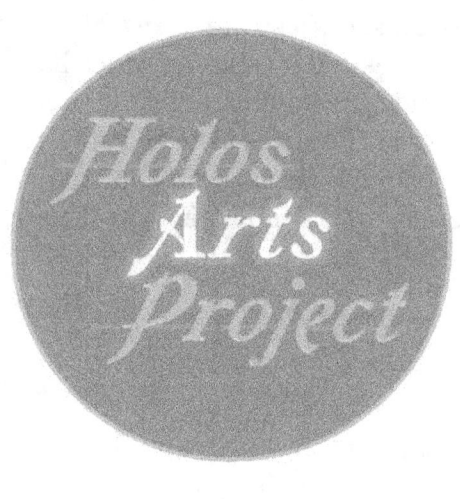

CONTENTS

Introduction 9

Chapter 1.
The Fundamentals of Reincarnation . . 13

Chapter 2.
Akashic Records: Accessing the Book of your Soul . 17

Chapter 3.
Healing through Past Life Therapy . . 22

Chapter 4.
Preparing for self-exploration . . . 26

Chapter 5.
Self-knowledge and internal preparation . . 29

Chapter 6.
Past Life Regression 34

Chapter 7.
Meditation and self-regression . . . 41

Chapter 8.
Overcoming Blocks and Fears . . . 44

Chapter 9.
Exploring the past:
deepening the study of a previous life . . 51

Chapter 10.
Themes and Patterns Throughout Previous Lives . 57

Chapter 11.
Karmic Connections:
Interpersonal Relationships Across Time . . 60

Chapter 12.
Inheriting Gifts from the Past:
Awakening Your Innate Talents . . . 63

Chapter 13.
Exploring Diverse Lives and Past Cultures . . 66

Chapter 14.
Anne's Journey: A Mosaic of Past Lives . . 69

Chapter 15.
*The Importance of Forgiveness and Self-Compassion
in the study of past lives.* 71

Chapter 16.
Exploring Future Lives: A glimpse of what can be . 73

Chapter 17.
Guided Meditation, Exploring Your Future Life . 76

Chapter 18.
*My personal experience during the exploration
of the period between lives* 79

Chapter 19.
Healing at the Collective Level . . . 88

Chapter 20.
*Integrating the Consciousness of the
Immortality of the Soul* 91

Chapter 21.
*Conclusions:
Embracing the Fabric of Our Past Histories* . 94

Introduction

Welcome to this fascinating journey towards self-knowledge through the exploration of your past lives. My name is Isis Estrada, and I am pleased to accompany you on this journey towards the discovery of your previous experiences, uncovering the enigmas of reincarnation. As a specialist in past life therapy, I have had the privilege of guiding countless individuals in their inner search, and it is with great empathy and warm gratitude that I invite you to explore this mysterious and revealing path towards understanding your deeper self.

The notion of reincarnation has existed throughout human history and has been addressed by various cultures and spiritual traditions. The essence of this belief holds that the soul is eternal and transcends physical death, being reborn in new bodies and contexts throughout multiple incarnations. It is a perspective that invites us to consider life as an infinite cycle of learning and evolution, and to see each existence as an opportunity to grow and expand as spiritual beings.

The idea of past lives suggests that our present experiences are intricately connected to the events and lessons we have experienced in the past. By exploring these previous lives, we can unravel recurring patterns, understand complex relationships and access ancient wisdom that still resides deep within us.

What do past lives tell us about ourselves? Imagine a mighty river, flowing from the past into the present and extending into the future. In each of its waters are the impressions, experiences and learnings of each of our lives. By diving into the depths of this river, we gain a broader and deeper vision of who we are in our purest essence. A canvas painted with the colors of our virtues, passions, fears and challenges is revealed.

Each stroke on that cosmic canvas connects us to the evolutionary narrative of our being, allowing us to better understand the meaning of our existence, but above all, and the purpose of our present events.

The main objective of this book is to open a portal to a fascinating and enriching world: the world of past lives. My intention is to provide you with the tools and guidance necessary to immerse yourself in the exploration of your previous existences, with the confidence and support necessary to discover and understand the lessons that still resonate in your soul. Throughout these pages, you will find techniques and exercises designed to help you remember your past lives and discover the wisdom hidden in each experience.

But beyond being a simple compilation of techniques, this book is an invitation for you to embark on a journey of self-discovery. Through past life therapy, you will confront unknown aspects of your being, and immerse yourself in an ocean of memories and emotions that will invite you to heal, grow and evolve. Here, my focus is to offer you a safe and compassionate space where you can face your fears and limitations and embrace your hidden gifts and strengths.

As you go through these pages, you will find personal examples that I share with the intention of illustrating the powerful transformation that past life therapy can trigger. These examples are a window into my own journey, a testament to how my past life exploration has been a beacon of light in my own spiritual and emotional evolution. Through these personal accounts, I trust that you will feel accompanied on your journey, knowing that you are not alone in your quest.

My path to understanding reincarnation began in adolescence when a series of vivid and recurring dreams connected me to times and places that defied the understanding of my rational mind. These experiences led me to investigate the possibility that our souls had lived before in different times and circumstances. My curiosity led me to study various philosophies and religions that addressed the concept of reincarnation and the notion of the immortality of the soul. However, it was in past life therapy that I found a profound and transformative avenue of exploration. My motivation as a therapist led me to become certified by The American Hypnosis Association, and to open my practice, where I have seen a large number of patients for over a decade. Through this valuable therapeutic tool, I was able to help individuals heal wounds rooted in past experiences, freeing their potential to live a fuller and more conscious present life.

In each chapter, I encourage you to keep a personal journal, recording your impressions, emotions and reflections as you progress through the book. This journal will become your faithful companion and keeper of your discoveries, allowing you to track your progress and relive key moments in your journey. The journal will be a sacred space where you can release your deepest thoughts and provide a haven for your emotions to flow freely.

It is important to mention that this book does not seek to demonstrate the objective veracity of reincarnation, but rather, to open a space for reflection and self-discovery. Regardless of your personal beliefs, I invite you to adopt an open-minded and receptive posture, allowing your intuition and inner wisdom to be your guides on this journey.

I also want to clarify that in this book when I mention cases that I have treated because they are relevant to the subject, the identity of my patients has been preserved, so I will be using fictitious names to fulfill that purpose.

This book is a course in the full extent of the word, which follows the world standards of the subject, and is accredited by The International Guild of Complementary Therapists (IGCT), from England. Anyone who has completed the course can request their diploma of completion, personalized with name and date, which is issued by the Centro de Terapias Alternativas Sendero Místico, in Mexico City, of which I am the general director. In the last section of the book, I give more extensive explanations on how to request the diploma.

Past life therapy is a profound and transformative tool that can open the doors of our past to illuminate the present and the future. I am excited to have you join me on this wonderful path of discovery, and hope that through these pages you will find the wisdom and healing you long for on your path to wholeness and spiritual growth.

With gratitude and expectation,
Isis Estrada.

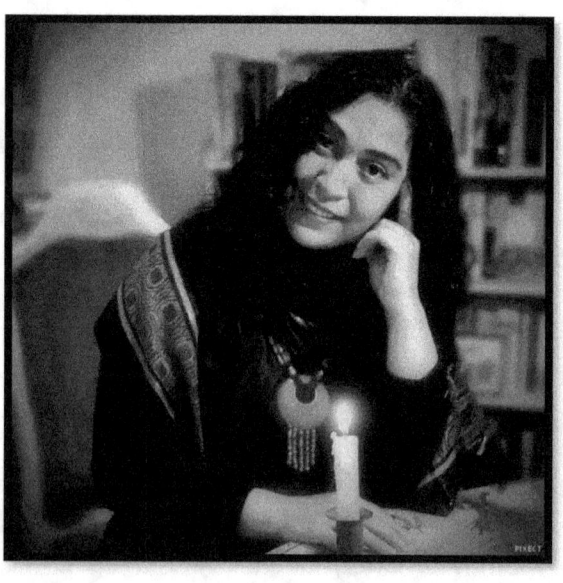

Chapter 1.

The Fundamentals of Reincarnation

Belief in reincarnation is a concept that has been deeply rooted in various cultures and religions over the centuries. The origins of this belief can be traced back to the most ancient civilizations, such as the ancient religious traditions of India and Egypt. In ancient Hindu culture, for example, there is the notion of "samsara," the eternal cycle of birth, death and rebirth. According to this belief, the soul or "atman" reincarnates again and again in different physical bodies, with the purpose of learning and evolving spiritually. Hindu sacred texts, such as the Upanishads and the Bhagavad Gita, have left a valuable legacy that delves into this subject.

In Egypt, belief in life after death and reincarnation was a central pillar of religion and spirituality. The ancient Egyptians practiced complex funerary rituals and buried their dead with treasures and objects they believed would be needed in their next life. Belief in reincarnation was also found in Greek and Roman cultures, and some classical philosophers such as Pythagoras and Plato held the idea that the soul is immortal and goes through multiple existences.

In the Middle Ages, belief in reincarnation was questioned by certain religious institutions, but it never completely vanished. Some mystics and philosophers, such as Plotinus and Origen, continued to explore and promote this notion. Eventually, the expansion of thought and freethought in the modern era allowed for a resurgence of belief in reincarnation,

As we moved into the modern era, belief in reincarnation did not disappear, but found new forms of expression. In the late

19th and early 20th centuries, spiritualism gained popularity in Europe and the United States, and attempts were made to communicate with the spirits of deceased loved ones. Through channeling and hypnosis, information about past lives emerged that inspired researchers and psychotherapists to further explore this phenomenon.

The emergence of clinical hypnosis in the late 19th century provided a powerful tool for exploring past lives. Pioneers such as French psychiatrist Pierre Janet and Swiss psychologist Carl Gustav Jung used hypnosis and regression techniques to help their patients release traumas and conflicts rooted in past life experiences.

In more recent years, past life therapy has become an approach increasingly used by therapists and mental health professionals. Documented case studies, such as that of psychiatrist Brian L. Weiss with his famous patient "Catherine" in his book "Many Lives, Many Masters," have sparked increased interest in the subject. Catherine, under hypnosis, vividly described past life experiences that, when explored, led to the resolution of her emotional problems in the present life.

In addition to case studies, scientific research has also shed light on the phenomenon of past lives. Research on cellular memory and epigenetics has revealed possible biological mechanisms that could explain how certain past life experiences or traumas could be passed down through the generations.

To understand the phenomenon of reincarnation, it is essential to explore the concept of the soul and its journey through different lifetimes. If we consider the soul as an eternal and spiritual entity, then reincarnation represents an opportunity for constant growth and evolution. Each life offers unique lessons and challenges that contribute to the development of the soul in its quest for wisdom and love.

In my own experience as a past life therapist, I have had the privilege of accompanying numerous people on regressive journeys through time. One such remarkable experience was with a man named Miguel (not his real name), who came to me seeking answers to his recurring nightmares and unexplained phobias. Under hypnosis, Miguel was transported to a past life as a soldier in a 19th century battle. By remembering and releasing the traumas of that previous life, the phobias and nightmares in his present life gradually dissipated, and his sense of inner peace was strengthened.

The concept of karma, originating in the Dharmic traditions of India, is closely linked to the belief in reincarnation. Karma refers to the law of cause and effect, where actions and decisions in a past life have repercussions in future lives. In other words, our present actions are the result of our past actions and, in turn, will influence our future lives. While some interpret karma as a punitive force, others see it as an opportunity for spiritual growth and evolution. For example, a person who has caused pain to others in a past life may experience similar situations in his or her current life as an opportunity to learn empathy and compassion. By recognizing and redeeming these lessons, the way is paved for the evolution of the soul toward greater understanding and wisdom.

A poignant illustration of karma was revealed during a past-life therapy session with a woman named Cinthia (not her real name). Under hypnosis, Cinthia relived a past life as a healer in a small village. During that life, she had helped many people with her abilities, but she had also experienced persecution and judgment by others who considered her a witch. In the present life, Cinthia had developed a deep fear of expressing her gifts and talents, which was limiting her personal and spiritual development. By becoming aware of this karmic connection, Cinthia was able to release her fears and embrace her healing potential with renewed confidence. Now, she is an alternative therapist and sees patients in a city in Latin America.

In this first chapter, we have addressed the historical and cultural background of the belief in reincarnation, as well as modern evidence and studies that have supported this notion over time. We explored the concept of the soul and how it goes through different lifetimes for spiritual growth, and how karma influences our journey through multiple existences. I hope your curiosity and desire to discover more about your own lives and how they can influence your present life has been awakened.

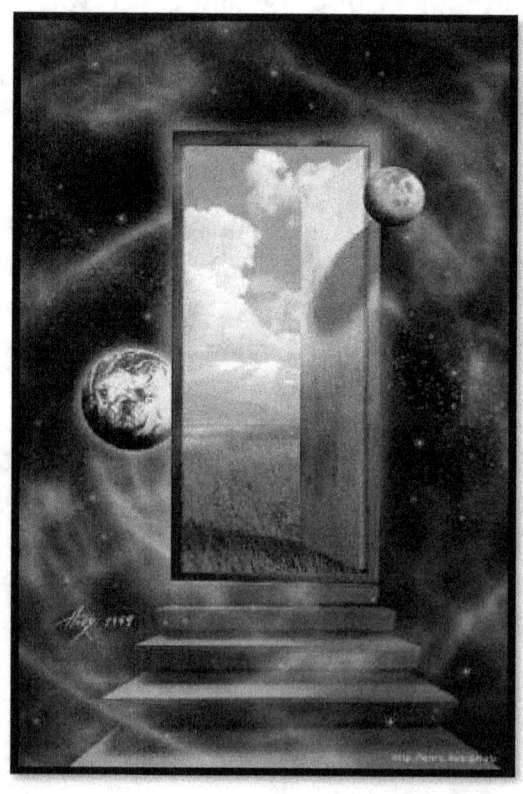

Chapter 2.

Akashic Records:
Accessing the book of your Soul

Dear reader, in this fascinating chapter, we will dive into the concept of the Akashic Records, a mystical and profound essence that holds the history of your past lives. The Akashic Records represent a vast library of the soul, which houses the information of all our past, present and future experiences. Through connection with these archives, we can gain valuable insights that will help us in our journey of self-knowledge and spiritual evolution.

Concept of the Akashic Records:

The Akashic Records, also known as the Book of Life or the Memory of the Universe, is an ancient belief in the existence of an energy field that contains all the experiences and events that have occurred since the beginning of time. This notion has been part of various spiritual and philosophical traditions throughout history. The term "Akasha" comes from Sanskrit and translates as "ether" or "primordial substance". According to this view, each soul has its own akashic record, which is unique and sacred, and is intimately linked to that soul's purpose and evolution. The akashic records are like an immense field of energetic information, where every event, emotion and thought leaves an eternal imprint.

Historical Context

The concept of the Akashic Records has been part of spiritual wisdom for millennia. In ancient Hindu culture, the Akasha is mentioned as the ethereal substance that permeates the universe. In the esoteric traditions of ancient Egypt, there was a belief in a "Book of Life" where the deeds of each individual were recorded. Likewise, the idea of the Akashic records has been transmitted through different philosophies and religions, such as Buddhism, Hermeticism and Theosophy.

In the 19th century, the influential figure of Helena Petrovna Blavatsky emerged on the spiritual and philosophical scene, leaving a profound mark on the way the Western world perceived esoteric and mystical concepts. Born in Ekaterinoslav, Russia, in 1831, Blavatsky spent much of her life traveling and exploring diverse traditions and cultures, which led her to acquire a vast and eclectic knowledge.

It was in 1875 when Blavatsky and Colonel Henry Steel Olcott founded the Theosophical Society in New York, with the aim of disseminating and exploring spiritual and philosophical teachings from around the world. Theosophy, as a movement, advocated the idea of a universal esoteric wisdom that was rooted in ancient traditions and that could provide a deeper understanding of the universe and the human being.

It was within this atmosphere of spiritual exploration that Helena Blavatsky introduced the notion of the Akashic Records to the West. Drawing on Eastern teachings and the mystical traditions of antiquity, Blavatsky described the Akashic records as an "indelible astral chart of all things that have been."

Blavatsky held that the akashic records could be accessed through spiritual perception and that human beings had the innate capacity to connect with them. For her, the akasha was the eternal link between man and the divine, and through its access, the individual could gain a deeper understanding of his or her spiritual nature and purpose in existence.

Accessing the Akashic records requires an opening of the mind and a connection with the heart. There is no single formula for reaching this spiritual dimension, but some common practices can help facilitate access to this profound wisdom:

Meditation and Visualization

Meditation is a powerful tool for calming the mind and raising consciousness. Through meditation focused on the Akashic records, you can open yourself to the perception of images, sensations or intuitions related to your past lives. You can begin by imagining a cosmic library, visualizing a sacred book that contains all the information about your previous lives. Practice this meditation regularly to strengthen your connection with this spiritual dimension.

Guided Akashic Records

In some cases, people may find it helpful to receive guidance from a therapist or akashic record specialist. These facilitators are trained to help you access your records and can provide a more structured and safe experience for those who are just beginning to explore this facet of themselves.

Intuition and Dreams

Our intuition can be a gateway to the wisdom of our Akashic records. Pay attention to hunches, dreams and synchronicities that manifest in your life, as they may contain significant messages about your past lives. Keep a journal to record these events and reflect on their possible connection to your previous experiences.

Exercises to start connecting with your Akashic Records

Now, I present you with a practical exercise that will help you establish a first meaningful connection with your Akashic records.

Exercise 1: Guided Meditation: The Letter of the Soul

To begin this powerful meditation, find a quiet space where you can be comfortable and free from distractions. Sit down with a sheet of paper and a pen within reach. Gently close your eyes and begin to breathe deeply, calmly inhaling and exhaling. Feel your body relax with each breath.

Now visualize a golden light shining brightly around you, enveloping you in its warm energy. This light represents the love and wisdom of the universe, which accompanies you on this journey into your past lives. Feel safe and protected by this divine light that will guide you in your quest for self-knowledge.

Now, with your mind focused on the purpose of this meditation, ask the universe to reveal to you a relevant teaching from a past life that may benefit you in your present. Open your heart to the possibility of receiving answers and deep insights.

With your eyes gently open, take the pen in your hand and place it on the blank paper. Allow yourself to feel the connection between the pen and your inner self, as if they were an extension of your soul.

Without judging or censoring your thoughts, allow yourself to flow in the act of writing. Let the words emerge from the depths of your being, as if you were channeling the wisdom of your past lives. Don't worry about grammar or structure; what is important is the sincerity and authenticity of your words.

As you write, pay attention to any images, words or emotions that arise in your mind. Allow yourself to become immersed in the experience, as if you were living a movie with image, sound, sensations, movement. Keep your mind open and receptive to what may arise.

Don't rush this process. Take your time to explore and reflect on what you are writing. If you encounter obstacles or roadblocks, just breathe and move on. Sometimes the deepest treasures lie beyond our first impressions.

Keep writing until you feel you have expressed everything you need to. This act of self-expression can be both liberating and revealing. When you feel you have reached a point of conclusion, take one last look at your words and thank the universe for the wisdom that has been revealed to you.

Now, close your eyes again and bring your attention to your heart. Feel how the energy of your written words infuses your being, integrating into your present self and enriching your present experience.

With gratitude in your heart, thank the universe for this valuable meditation and for the wisdom you have received. Recognize that you are connected to an eternal stream of knowledge and love that transcends time and space.

When you feel ready, gently open your eyes and return to the present. Keep your soul card in a special place, so that you can return to it in moments of reflection and self-knowledge.

Remember that this meditation can be repeated as many times as you wish, each time deepening your knowledge of your past lives and enriching your spiritual growth in the present.

For a recorded version of this meditation, access the Holos Arts Project YouTube channel and search for "Guided Meditation: The Letter of the Soul".

Chapter 3.

Healing through Past Life Therapy

Past Life Therapy (PLT) has proven to be a powerful tool in the field of psychotherapy, providing a unique and profound perspective for emotional and spiritual healing. Through the exploration of our past lives, we can delve into the depths of our psyche, unveiling the hidden mysteries that influence our current reality. The fundamental idea behind this therapy lies in the belief in reincarnation, which suggests that our souls have experienced multiple lives and that the unresolved experiences and emotions of those past lives can manifest in our current life.

Imagine that our present existence is only a small part of a vast canvas that spans time and space. Each life we have lived is woven into this great cosmic canvas, creating subtle patterns and connections that affect the way we are in the present. By delving into the past, we not only access specific episodes from past lives, but also gain a deeper understanding of our soul's ongoing evolution. It is as if we unlock doors to hidden chambers within ourselves, revealing the wisdom and emotional wounds that have shaped our current personality and behaviors.

At the heart of Past Life Therapy lies the notion that our soul is in constant search for balance and learning. By facing the unresolved challenges of past lives, we open ourselves to the possibility of healing deep-seated emotional wounds, freeing us from the weight of the past and allowing us to move toward greater wholeness in our present life.

In this chapter, we will closely explore four fascinating case studies that illustrate the transformative impact of Past Life

Therapy on individuals. Through these narratives, we will dive into the experiences of those who have experienced significant changes in their emotional and spiritual well-being through PLT.

Furthermore, it is crucial to note that Past Life Therapy is not an isolated approach but can complement and enrich other forms of therapy. When combined with traditional therapies, such as cognitive-behavioral therapy or Gestalt therapy, PLT broadens the understanding of the underlying patterns that affect the individual's behavior and emotions in the present. This allows for a more holistic and deeper approach to healing and personal growth.

1. Healing the deep fear: The case of Alejandra (not her real name) - May 30, 2002.

Alejandra, 32, had struggled for years with an unexplained phobia of water. She couldn't even go near a pool without going into a state of panic. In her first Past Life Therapy session, Alejandra experienced a regression that took her back to a past life as a young sailor who tragically drowned during a shipwreck. Through this experience, she was able to understand that her current phobia was rooted in that traumatic past life. Working with this information, Alejandra began to release her deep-seated fear of water and was eventually able to swim in a pool without feeling terror. PLT allowed her to heal emotions that were trapped over time and release them in the present.

2. Releasing Repetitive Patterns: The Case of Daniel (not his real name) - September 15, 2008.

Daniel, 45, was stuck in a repetitive cycle of failed relationships and financial problems. In his PLT regressions, he discovered connections to several previous lives where he had experienced similar situations. In one past life, he was a monk who had taken a vow of poverty and, in another, a merchant who had suffered bankruptcy. These repetitive patterns were hindering his growth in his current life. By recognizing and understanding these connections, Daniel was able to free himself from negative patterns and make more conscious and empowered choices in his present life.

3. Healing Unresolved Trauma: The Case of Olivia (not her real name) - November 10, 2012.

Olivia, 38, suffered from recurrent anxiety attacks with no apparent cause. In PLT, she traced back to a past life where she witnessed a devastating fire that caused her deep emotional trauma. Through therapy, she was able to confront and release the repressed emotions associated with that traumatic event. The release of that emotional weight allowed Olivia to experience significant improvement in her anxiety attacks and she found a sense of inner peace that she had been seeking for a long time.

4. Complementing other therapies: the case of Samuel (not his real name) - January 5, 2018.

Samuel, 50, had been attending traditional therapy for years to address his depression and low self-esteem. While he found some relief in those sessions, he felt there were underlying unresolved issues. With Past Life Therapy, Samuel discovered a past life in which he had been rejected by his family for his choice of partner. This experience had left a deep mark on his self-esteem and negatively affected his current life. By integrating PLT with his traditional therapy, Samuel was able to delve deeper into the roots of his low self-esteem and work to transform his negative beliefs, finding greater understanding and love for himself.

Past Life Therapy has been shown to be a valuable tool for emotional and spiritual healing, complementing and empowering other forms of therapy. By allowing us to explore the deeper roots of our current challenges, we can release traumas and limiting patterns that affect us in the present. PLT not only offers a more complete understanding of ourselves, but also gives us the opportunity to heal and grow in a meaningful way.

I hope these case studies have shed light on the transformative potential of knowing our past lives. Remember that each individual is unique, and the PLT experience may vary. It is always important to seek out a trained and experienced therapist to guide this journey of self-discovery.

Chapter 4.

Preparing for Exploration

We will delve into the fundamental preparation to begin our process of past life exploration. We will address the importance of keeping an open mind and the essential role of intuition in this fascinating journey. In addition, we will dive into creating the right space and environment for our exploration sessions, as well as the relevance of keeping a journal to record our experiences. With passion and empathy, I invite you to dive into this chapter and prepare to enter the mysterious world of our past lives.

Understanding the importance of open-mindedness and intuition:

When we embark on the journey of exploring our past lives, it is essential that we keep an open and flexible mind. We must be willing to question our previous beliefs and assumptions, allowing us to embrace new perspectives and understand the vastness of time and the soul. Open-mindedness allows us to receive the revelations of our past experiences without filters or judgments, which will make it easier for us to integrate these experiences with our present.

Intuition plays a prominent role in this process. It is the internal compass that will guide us to the areas of our past that require our attention. Through intuition, we can access hidden memories and information that manifest as sensations, images or emotions. It is important to learn to trust our intuition and to recognize the signals it indicates to us. In doing so, we allow ourselves to discover and understand more deeply the lessons learned in previous lives and how they impact our present life.

Preparing the appropriate space and environment for the exploration sessions:

Creating a space conducive to past life exploration sessions is fundamental in our process of self-knowledge. A calm and serene environment helps us to concentrate and connect with our deepest essence. Here are some tips for preparing such a space:

1. Selecting the place: Let's look for a place where we can be in peace and without interruptions during our sessions. It can be a quiet room in our house or a corner in nature that inspires tranquility and connection.
2. Comforting elements: Let's add elements that bring us comfort and tranquility. Candles, incense, stones, crystals or meaningful images can help us create an environment conducive to exploration.
3. Relaxing music: Let's listen to soft and relaxing music, which helps us to relax and get into a receptive state of mind.
4. Elimination of distractions: Let's turn off our electronic devices and any other source of distraction that may disrupt our focus.

Tips for keeping a journal and recording experiences:

Keeping a journal of our past life exploration experiences is essential for keeping an accurate record of our discoveries and progress. Here are some recommendations for keeping an effective journal:

1. Immediate recording: As soon as you finish a scanning session, write down all relevant details while they are still fresh in your mind. Even seemingly insignificant details can reveal valuable information later.

2. Sensory and emotional details: Describe not only what we saw, but also what we felt, heard and experienced emotionally during the session. These details can provide a more complete understanding of our past experiences.

3. Synchronicities: Let us pay attention to synchronicities and coincidences that may occur in our lives after an exploration session. These events may be related to our past discoveries and will help us integrate them with our present reality.

4. Patterns and lessons: As we move forward on our journey, let's look for recurring patterns or lessons that present themselves throughout our past lives. These patterns can offer deeper insight into the issues we are meant to address and heal in this lifetime.

By keeping a diary and recording our experiences, we will be able to track our progress and evolution.

Chapter 5.

Self-knowledge and Internal Preparation

In the fascinating journey of discovering our past lives, self-knowledge and inner preparation play a fundamental role. Before embarking on the exploration of our ancestral memories, it is crucial that we immerse ourselves in a process of deep and honest self-reflection. This chapter is designed to guide you through this crucial stage, enabling you to identify clear goals and key questions for your journey of self-exploration.

The importance of self-reflection:
Self-reflection is a powerful tool that helps us to understand our deepest essence, our personality and how we have become who we are today. It is a journey into our inner self, where we can examine our emotions, behaviors and ingrained beliefs. By knowing and accepting our strengths and weaknesses, we can approach our past life search with an open and receptive mindset.

Self-knowledge is the foundation upon which we will build our journey of discovery. By knowing our own tendencies, patterns and fears, we will be able to discern between those aspects of our personality that are inherent to our essence and those that may be influenced by our past lives. Self-reflection also provides us with the opportunity to release emotional burdens and blocks that may arise during the exploration process.

Identification of objectives and key questions:
Before delving into the vast ocean of our past lives, it is important to establish clear objectives for our quest. What do we hope to achieve with this journey of self-knowledge? Are we

seeking to understand and heal past traumas, discover hidden talents, or unlock the purpose of our current existence? Each individual may have different motivations for embarking on this path, and it is essential to define them honestly.

To help you identify your objectives, consider the following questions:

1. What recurring issues or problems do I face in my life today that could be linked to past experiences?
2. What aspects of my personality do I feel I cannot fully explain from my current life history?
3. Are there unexplained talents, skills or interests that intrigue me?
4. What emotional challenges or deep fears seem to persist in my life for no apparent reason?
5. Do you experience a strong connection to a particular historical period or place?
6. Have I met people who immediately arouse my affection or empathy, as if I had known them for many years?

Learning to connect with our intuition and inner guidance:

Once we have established our goals, it is time to develop a deeper connection with our intuition and inner guidance. Our inner self is a valuable and wise resource that can provide us with valuable insights into our past lives.

Meditation and mindfulness practice are effective tools for calming the mind and opening channels to our deepest self. By taking time for quiet reflection, we can access memories and sensations that would otherwise remain hidden. Meditation also helps us to increase our ability to receive intuitive messages that can direct us on our journey of self-exploration.

Another tool for connecting with our inner guidance is to keep a dream journal. Dreams often act as doorways to deeper dimensions of our psyche and recording them can reveal connections to our past lives. Pay special attention to recurring dreams or those that evoke intense emotions, as they may be related to ancestral memories.

Also, the practice of self-hypnosis can facilitate access to our oldest mental archives. Through guided relaxation and visualization techniques, we can explore our subconscious and unlock memories that lie deep within our mind.

It is essential to approach the process of connecting with our intuition and inner guidance with patience and openness. Not all memories will be clear and vivid at first, and it may take time to decipher the messages we receive.

The journey of discovering our past lives is an exciting adventure that invites us to dive into the depths of our being. Self-reflection and self-knowledge form the solid basis for this quest, and the connection with our intuition and inner guidance will take us by the hand through the intricate labyrinth of our past existences.

I encourage you to try the following short self-hypnosis exercise, to start "warming up" in the exploration of your past lives.

Self-Hypnosis: Brief Journey to a Past Life.

Welcome to this guided meditation to explore a brief but vivid scene from a past life. Before you begin, make sure you are in a quiet, comfortable place where you will not be interrupted. Sit or lie down in a relaxed position, gently closing your eyes, and take several deep breaths to center and calm your mind.

Breathe deeply, inhaling slowly through your nose and exhaling gently through your mouth. Feel the air fill your lungs and the tension release with each exhalation. Allow your body to relax completely, feeling it sink into a deep serenity and inner peace.

Now, bring your attention to your own mind. Visualize a staircase in front of you, a beautiful staircase descending into the depths of your being. This staircase represents access to your subconscious, where the memories of your past lives reside.

Begin to descend the staircase calmly and confidently, taking each step with confidence. As you descend, feel your mind clear and free of any external distractions. Each step you take takes you deeper within, bringing you closer to the source of your ancient wisdom.

You reach the last step and find yourself in a quiet and peaceful place in your subconscious. Here, in this sacred space, you can explore a past life. As you look around you, you will notice a door in front of you. This door leads to the scene you wish to visualize. You may have a question or intention in mind before you open the door, such as "Show me a scene from a past life relevant to my current purpose" or "I want to see a lesson I need to learn".

With determination and confidence, open the door and step into the scene before you. You may find yourself in a natural landscape, in an ancient city, or in an everyday scene of life in the past. Don't worry if at first you see only fragments or shadows, clarity will come with practice and patience.

Observe your surroundings, pay attention to details, colors, smells and sensations. What kind of clothes are you wearing? What emotions are you feeling at this moment? You can interact with the characters or simply be an observer. Allow yourself to become completely immersed in the scene, without judgment or expectations, just allowing the story to unfold before your eyes.

As you become more and more immersed in the scene, you may begin to notice important information about that past life. What is your role in this life? What is your name? What important events occurred in this time period? Let the information flow to you, trust your intuition and the wisdom of your subconscious.

If at any time you feel discomfort or tension, remember that you are in control and can return to the staircase at any time. This meditation should be a liberating and healing experience, so feel free to modify the scene or leave it if you wish.

Now, it is time to end this exploration. Thank your subconscious for revealing this scene to you and, with gratitude, step back and close the door. Slowly begin to ascend the staircase, climbing each step calmly and taking with you the insights gained in this meditation.

Return to your present space, feeling how your body is comfortably sitting or lying down, breathing softly and calmly. Open your eyes when you are ready and allow a moment to reconnect with the environment around you.

Remember that this meditation is only the beginning. As you continue to practice self-hypnosis and the exploration of your ancestral memories, you will experience greater clarity and connection to your deeper self. Allow these memories to guide you on your path to self-knowledge and spiritual growth.

To listen to a recorded version of this guided self-hypnosis, search the Holos Arts Project YouTube channel for the video called "Self-Hypnosis: Brief Journey to a Past Life."

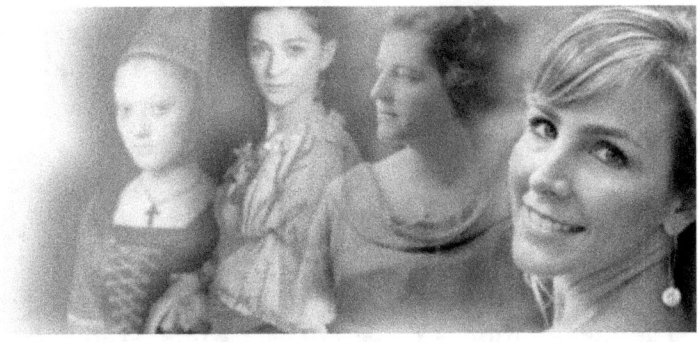

Chapter 6.

Past Life Regression

The quest for knowledge that transcends the boundaries of time and space has captivated the human mind over the centuries. In the vast tapestry of existence, our past lives present themselves as interwoven threads that have contributed to weave the fabric of our current incarnation. Past life regression stands as an invaluable tool in this exploration of the self, allowing us to delve into the depths of our previous experiences and ultimately access a greater understanding of our purpose and evolution.

Diverse Exploration Trails

Past life regression is a process that can be approached through a variety of techniques, each with its own uniqueness and focus. Among the most notable are hypnotic regression, deep meditation and past life therapy. Each of these paths offers a different means of achieving the same goal: the unraveling of the veils that conceal memories of previous existences.

Hypnotic regression, in particular, has been a vehicle of choice for many spiritual seekers. Guided by an experienced therapist, individuals can immerse themselves in an altered state of consciousness that facilitates access to their deepest memories. Through relaxation and suggestion, a window into the distant past is opened, allowing a review of events and circumstances that shaped previous stages of their life trajectory.

Ethical Considerations and Wise Precautions

The exploration of past lives, while stimulating and revealing, must be approached with caution and sensitivity. It is vital that those undertaking this journey understand the sensitive nature of these memories and how they can impact their emotional and mental well-being. The connection to past traumatic events can elicit intense reactions, underscoring the importance of having the support of a competent therapist.

It is crucial to recognize that while past life regression can bring clarity and healing, it can also expose us to unexpected challenges. Emotions and perceptions can be intense, and it is critical to establish emotional boundaries to safeguard our psychological stability. The guidance of an experienced and empathic therapist can be a beacon on this journey, providing the support needed to navigate often uncharted emotional waters.

What ethical considerations and precautions should be taken into account for safe exploration? Past life regression is a personal and intimate experience that involves accessing sensitive and potentially traumatic information. Therefore, some ethical principles must be respected and some precautionary measures must be taken to avoid unnecessary risk or harm. Some of these principles and measures are:

Informed consent: This is the right of every person to receive clear and truthful information about the method, objectives, benefits, risks and alternatives of past life regression before deciding whether or not to participate in it. Informed consent must be voluntary, free and revocable at any time.

Respect for autonomy: This is the right of every person to freely choose whether or not to perform a past life regression, as well as to determine the pace, depth and scope of their exploration. Respect for autonomy implies not pressuring, manipulating, inducing or coercing anyone to perform a past life regression against their will or interest.

Confidentiality: It is the duty of any person who performs or attends a past life regression to keep secret the information that is revealed during the regression, unless there is an express consent of the interested party or a legal obligation that prevents it. Confidentiality implies not disclosing, sharing, publishing or using the information obtained for purposes other than those previously agreed upon.

Safety: It is the responsibility of every person who performs or attends a past life regression to ensure the proper conditions for a safe and positive experience. Safety involves choosing an appropriate method, a competent practitioner, a comfortable and peaceful environment, and sufficient time for the preparation, conduct and integration of the past life regression.

Guided hypnotic regression exercise to a past life

Next, I propose a practical exercise for you to experience a guided hypnotic regression to a past life. For this, you will need a quiet place where you will not be disturbed, a headset and a recording with the instructions I will give you. I recommend that you do this exercise with the help of a friend or family member who can accompany you and assist you in case you need it. I also suggest that you have a notebook and pen at hand so that you can write down your impressions after the regression.

Before you begin, make sure you are in a state of physical and mental relaxation. Take several deep breaths and release any tension or worries you may have. Feel comfortable and confident. Remember that you are about to go on a journey of self-knowledge and that you can control your experience at all times.

Now, put on your headphones and press play on the recording. Listen carefully to the instructions and follow the indications I will give you. Don't worry if you don't understand something or if you don't see anything at first.

Let your imagination and intuition guide you. Trust your subconscious memory and your inner guidance.

Ready? Let's get started!

Guided hypnotic regression to a past life.

Welcome to this guided past life regression meditation. This practice will allow you to access the memories of your subconscious mind, where your past life experiences are stored. These experiences can have an impact on your current life, both positive and negative, and by remembering them you will be able to better understand who you are, what you are here to do and what you need to heal.

Now, close your eyes and breathe deeply. Breathe in through your nose and out through your mouth, slowly and calmly. Feel the air flow in and out of your body, filling you with energy and peace. With each breath, release any tension or stress you may have. Let your body relax completely, from head to toe.

Now, imagine that you are in a safe and beautiful place, where you feel happy and calm. It can be a real or imaginary place, the important thing is that it is a place that you like and that inspires confidence. Observe the details of that place, the colors, the sounds, the aromas. Feel how that place envelops you with its love and protection.

In that place, there is a door that opens before you. It is a magical door, which will take you to one of your past lives. You don't have to be afraid or doubtful, just curious and open. Behind that door there is a treasure for you, valuable information that will help you on your way.

Approach the door and gently open it. On the other side is a staircase descending downward. Begin to descend the staircase, feeling each step take you deeper into your subconscious. Mentally count the rungs as you go down: ten, nine, eight, seven, six, five, four, three, two, one.

You have reached the top of the stairs. You are in a dark and silent corridor. You see nothing and hear nothing, you only feel your own presence. You know you are about to enter one of your past lives.

At the end of the hallway is another door. It is the door that connects you to your past life. Go to it and open it with determination.

When you open the door, you enter a scene from your past life. It is as if you are watching a movie of your own history. You can see what is going on around you, but you can also feel what you are feeling at that moment.

Look carefully at what you see: where are you? what time of year is it? what are you wearing? what are you doing? are there other people with you? what are they like? how do you relate to them?

Try to identify who you are in that past life: what is your name, your age, your gender, your profession, your personality, your dreams, your fears?

Pay attention also to how you feel: are you happy or sad? restless or nervous? satisfied or frustrated? in love or lonely?

Stay in that scene for as long as you need to absorb as much information as possible. Do not judge or analyze what you see or feel, just observe and experience.

When you think you've seen enough, exit that scene and return to the dark hallway. Close the door behind you and take a deep breath. You have returned to the present, but you have brought with you a memory of your past life.

Now, reflect on what you have seen and felt. What has struck you? What has surprised you? What has moved you? What has taught you?

Think about how that past life relates to your current life. Are there any similarities or differences? Are there any lessons or messages you can apply now? Are there any wounds or blockages you can heal?

Thank your subconscious mind for showing you that past life. Also thank your soul for having lived that experience. Recognize the value and purpose of each of your lives, and how they are all part of your evolution.

Now, return to the magical door that brought you here. Open it and climb the ladder, feeling each step lift you higher in your consciousness. Mentally count the steps as you climb: one, two, three, four, five, six, seven, eight, nine, ten.

You have arrived at the safe and beautiful place where you started. Feel how that place welcomes you with joy and pride. You have made a wonderful journey and have returned wiser and happier.

Take a deep breath and open your eyes. You have finished the guided past life regression meditation. I hope you have enjoyed this experience and learned something new about yourself. I invite you to write down what you have seen and felt on a piece of paper or in a journal, so that you can remember and reflect on it later.

Thank you for joining me in this meditation. I wish you the best in your path of self-knowledge and personal growth. See you next time. Namaste.

* * * *

When you finish the exercise, take a few minutes to come back to reality. Stretch your body, drink water, breathe deeply. Share your impressions with your companion or write them down in your notebook. Think about what you have learned about yourself and your current life.

I hope you found this exercise useful and interesting. Remember that you can repeat it as many times as you want, always with respect, caution and curiosity. Each past life regression is unique and unrepeatable and can offer you new perspectives and opportunities to grow as a person.

For a recorded version, go to the Holos Arts Project YouTube channel and search for it under the name: Guided Hypnotic Regression to a Past Life.

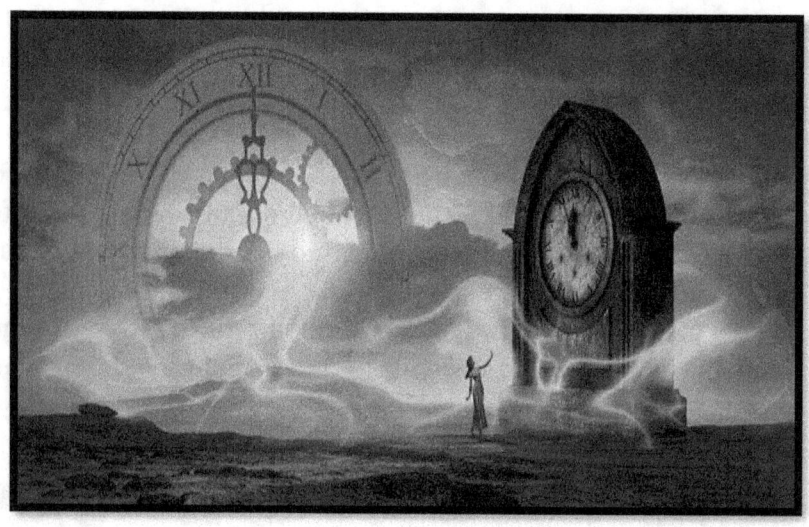

Chapter 7.
Meditation and Self-Regression

Meditation is an ancient practice that consists of focusing attention on an object, thought, sensation or breath in order to calm the mind and achieve a state of relaxation, awareness and harmony. Meditation has multiple benefits for physical, mental and emotional health, such as reducing stress, improving sleep, increasing creativity, strengthening the immune system and developing emotional intelligence.

In the vast and enigmatic realm of past life exploration, meditation emerges as an essential tool for unraveling the subtle threads that connect our present being with ancestral experiences. The art of remembering past lives through meditation is a journey of self-discovery and self-knowledge that allows us to glimpse into the hidden depths of our being, revealing the traces of ancient incarnations that shape our present existence.

Meditation, in its essence, is a contemplative practice that allows us to transcend the confines of the conscious mind and enter into the deepest realms of the psyche. Through concentration and mental focus, we open the doors to inner perception and clear the way to access the memory stored in the recesses of our soul. This conscious act of introspection gives us the opportunity to relive fragments of past experiences and unravel the karmic connections that bind us through time.

The technique of effectively meditating and remembering past lives is a discipline that requires patience, dedication and a deep commitment to self-discovery. Here, in this chapter, we will dive into the fundamental steps that will guide your journey to self-regression through meditation.

Technique for an Effective Meditation State.

Meditation is an ancient art that amalgamates mind, body and spirit in a dance of serenity and self-connection. Allow me to immerse you in the depths of this transcendental practice in a journey that will lead you to discover its nuances and secrets.

Begin by choosing a quiet, comfortable place to sit or lie down. Your posture should be upright and relaxed, allowing the energy to flow unhindered. Close your eyes gently, inviting introspection.

The breath, essential guide, connects you to the present. Direct your attention to the rhythmic flow of the breath. Observe how the air flows in and out, without forcing or disturbing. As your mind wanders, gently redirect it to this vital cadence.

Concentration, the gateway to depth, is based on a point of focus. It can be the breath, a mantra or a mental image. Hold on to this anchor, avoiding being swept away by the waves of thoughts. When you wander, without judgment, gently return.

Acceptance and patience, unwavering allies, accompany your journey. Thoughts and emotions will surface; let them be, do not cling to them or reject them. Acknowledge them and allow them to flow, like leaves in the river of your mind.

Unbiased observation, an internal compass, leads you to self-knowledge. Explore your thoughts without identifying with them. Visualize them as passing clouds in the vast sky of your being, fading in the breeze of time.

Consistency, the elixir of progress, cultivates daily practice. Set a schedule and commit to it. Over time, meditation becomes ingrained in your routine, unfolding its benefits in all aspects of your life.

Self-compassion, a healing nectar, envelops you in unconditional love. As you explore your inner self, areas of resistance and shadow will emerge. Embrace these facets with tenderness, recognizing that they are an integral part of your being.

The expansion of consciousness, an endless horizon, awakens you to deeper dimensions. Over time, meditation transcends the limits of the individual, connecting you with the universe in a cosmic dance of energy and consciousness.

In this meditative journey into past lives, remember that each experience is unique and personal. There is no rigid formula or pre-established outcome. The magic lies in opening your heart and mind to exploration, allowing you to unravel the mysteries of your existence over time. With consistent practice and a genuine willingness, meditation becomes a compass that guides your steps into the very fabric of your ancestral history.

Chapter 8.

Overcoming Blocks and Fears

In the previous chapters, we have seen how to access our past lives through different methods, such as hypnosis, meditation, dreams or synchronicities. We have learned to recognize the signs that we are connecting with a memory from another existence, and to interpret the meaning and purpose of those experiences. We have also explored the benefits that remembering our past lives can have for our personal and spiritual growth, such as healing traumas, understanding our relationships, expanding our consciousness or releasing our karma.

However, not everything is easy and simple in this process. Sometimes, we may encounter obstacles that prevent us from accessing our past lives, or that make it difficult for us to handle the information we receive. These obstacles can be of an internal or external nature and can have different forms and origins. Some examples are:

Emotional blocks: These are those feelings or emotions that prevent us from relaxing and opening ourselves to the experience of regression. They can be fears, doubts, anxiety, guilt, shame, anger, sadness, etc. These emotions can be related to our current life, to a past life, or both. They may arise before, during or after the regression.

Mental blocks: These are those thoughts or beliefs that limit or condition us when accessing our past lives. They can be prejudices, skepticism, rationalization, denial, confusion, distraction, etc. These thoughts can be influenced by our education, our culture, our religion or our personality. They can appear at any point in the process.

Physical blocks: These are those external factors that interfere with our ability to concentrate and relax. They can be noises, lights, temperatures, discomfort, hunger, thirst, sleep, pain, etc. These factors may depend on our environment, our state of health or our basic needs. They can occur before or during the regression.

These blocks can act individually or in combination and can vary in intensity and frequency according to each person and each situation. However, they all have something in common: they are a form of resistance of our ego to face the unknown, to what may pose a change or a threat to our identity or our security.

Therefore, it is important that we are aware of these blocks and that we learn to overcome them with patience and confidence. In this chapter I will offer you some techniques to help you release repressed emotions and overcome resistance. I will also give you some tips for dealing with difficult or traumatic experiences during regression.

Releasing repressed emotions

Emotions are an essential part of our being. They are what allow us to feel and express what we are and what we live. However, we often do not know how to manage our emotions properly. Sometimes we repress them because they are uncomfortable or unacceptable. Other times we project them onto other people or situations because we do not want to assume our responsibility. And sometimes we deny them because we are unable to recognize or accept them.

These attitudes can generate emotional blocks that prevent us from accessing our past lives or integrating them into our current life. That is why it is important that we learn to release our repressed emotions and express them in a healthy and constructive way.

One way to do this is through therapeutic writing. This technique consists of writing about our feelings and thoughts without censorship or judgment. The goal is to let what is inside us flow without worrying about form or content. All we need is a piece of paper and a pen (or a computer) and a space and time where we can be quiet and uninterrupted.

To practice therapeutic writing, you can follow these steps:

Choose a topic you want to write about. It can be something that worries you, that bothers you, that hurts you, that makes you happy, that excites you, etc. It can be related to your current life or to a past life that you have remembered or want to remember.

Write for about 15 to 20 minutes without stopping. Don't worry about spelling, grammar or coherence. Just write what you feel and think about your chosen topic. Don't criticize or judge yourself. Be honest and sincere with yourself.

When you finish writing, read what you have written and reflect on it. What emotions did you experience while writing? What did you learn about yourself? What can you do to improve your situation or solve your problem? What actions can you take to express your emotions in a positive way?

Keep what you have written or destroy it if you prefer. The important thing is that you have released what you had inside and that you have become aware of it.

Another way to release repressed emotions is through conscious breathing. This technique consists of paying attention to our breathing and modifying it according to our needs. The goal is to relax our body and mind and connect with our inner self. We only need a comfortable and quiet place where we can be sitting or lying down.

To practice conscious breathing, you can follow these steps:

Close your eyes and place one hand on your chest and one hand on your abdomen. Breathe deeply through your nose and exhale through your mouth. Feel your hands move in rhythm with your breathing. Do this for a few minutes until you feel calm and centered.

Now, focus your attention on an emotion that you want to release. It may be an emotion that you have felt recently or one that is associated with a past life. Identify where that emotion is located in your body: is it in your chest, stomach, throat, head...? What shape, color or temperature does it have? What name would you give it?

Then imagine that emotion dissolving with each inhalation and being expelled with each exhalation. Visualize how the air enters through your nose and reaches the place where the emotion is. Then, imagine how the air exits through your mouth taking the emotion with it. Repeat this process until you feel that the emotion is gone or reduced.

Finally, breathe normally and observe how you feel after releasing the emotion. What changes do you notice in your body, mind or mood? What message has that emotion left you? What can you do to prevent or manage that emotion in the future?

These are just two of the many techniques that exist to release repressed emotions. You can try others such as yoga, art, music, dance, sport, etc. The important thing is that you find the one that best suits you and your circumstances.

Overcoming resistance

Resistances are those attitudes or behaviors that prevent us from accessing our past lives or integrating them into our current life. They are a form of defense of our ego in the face of the unknown, the different or the threatening. Resistances can manifest themselves in various ways, such as:

- Denying the existence of past lives or their influence on our present life.
- Doubting the veracity or relevance of the information we receive during regression.

- Rationalizing or minimizing experiences in other existences.
- Becoming distracted or disconnected during the regression process.
- Avoiding or rejecting the implications or consequences of remembering our past lives.

These resistances can have different origins, such as:

- Fear of facing aspects of pain. We are not only a company with a strong or difficult personality, but also with a strong or difficult past.
- Lack of confidence in our ability or right to access our past lives.
- Incongruence between our current beliefs or values and those of our past lives.
- Negative influence from other people or society who discourage or criticize us for exploring our past lives.

These resistances can be conscious or unconscious and can vary in intensity and frequency according to each person and each situation. However, they all have something in common: they are a form of self-sabotage that prevents us from taking advantage of the potential and resources we have within ourselves.

Therefore, it is important that we are aware of these resistances and that we learn to overcome them with courage and determination. In this chapter I will offer you some techniques to help you overcome resistances. I will also give you some tips for dealing with difficult or traumatic experiences during regression.

Positive affirmation

One way to overcome resistance is through positive affirmation. This technique consists of repeating phrases or words that motivate, inspire or strengthen us. The goal is to reprogram our mind and change our negative thoughts for positive ones.

All we need is a piece of paper and a pen (or a computer) and a space and time where we can be quiet and uninterrupted.

To practice positive affirmation, you can follow these steps:

Choose a phrase or a word that you like and that makes you feel good. It can be something you have read, heard or made up. It can be related to your current life or to a past life you have remembered or would like to remember.

Write the phrase or word on a piece of paper and place it in a visible place where you can see it often. You can also write it on your computer or cell phone and put it as a wallpaper or reminder.

Repeat the phrase or word mentally or out loud every time you see it or remember it. Do it with conviction, enthusiasm and joy. Feel how that phrase or word fills you with energy, confidence and love.

When you finish repeating the phrase or word, be grateful for the message it has conveyed and the effect it has had on you. Recognize your value, your potential and your ability to access your past lives and integrate them into your present life.

Some examples of positive phrases or words are:

- I am able to remember my past lives and learn from them.
- My past lives are a source of wisdom, love and light.
- I accept and love myself as I am, with all my past and present experiences.
- I trust my intuition and inner guidance to explore my past lives.
- I am open to receive messages and lessons from my past lives.

Creative visualization

Another way to overcome resistance is through creative visualization. This technique consists of imagining scenes or situations that help us achieve our goals or solve our problems. The objective is to create an alternative reality in our mind that will drive us to act accordingly. We only need a comfortable and quiet place where we can be sitting or lying down.

To practice creative visualization, you can follow these steps:

Close your eyes and take a deep breath in through your nose and out through your mouth. Relax your body and mind and focus your attention on your goal or problem. It may be something you want to achieve, improve, change, solve, etc. It can be related to your current life or to some past life that you have remembered or want to remember.

Now, imagine a scene or a situation where you have achieved your goal or solved your problem. Visualize as many details as possible: the colors, the sounds, the smells, the sensations, the people, etc. Make it as realistic as possible, but also as positive as possible.

Next, imagine how it feels to have achieved your goal or solved your problem. What emotions do you experience? What thoughts do you have? What words do you say or hear? What actions do you take or receive? Feel how that scene or situation fills you with satisfaction, pride and happiness.

Finally, open your eyes and come back to reality. See how you feel after visualizing your success or solution. What change do you notice in your body, mind or mood? What steps can you take to make your visualization a reality? What resources or supports can you use to achieve it?

These are just two of the many techniques that exist to overcome resistance. You can try others such as meditation, prayer, coaching, therapy, etc. The important thing is that you find the one that best suits you and your circumstances.

Chapter 9.

Exploring the Past:
Deepening the Study of a Past Life

In the previous chapters, we have seen how to access our past life memories through regressive hypnosis, meditation, dreaming and other techniques. We have learned to identify the signs that tell us that we have lived before and to recognize the connections between our current experiences and those of other times. We have also discovered how our past lives influence our personality, our relationships, our talents, our fears and our challenges.

But it is not enough to remember our past lives. For this knowledge to be useful and beneficial to our spiritual growth, we must delve deeper into the study of a specific past life. Why choose just one life among the many we have had? Because each life has a purpose, a lesson and a message that we can apply to our present life. By focusing on a life that catches our attention or generates a strong emotion, we can explore its details and meaning with greater clarity and depth.

How to deepen the study of a previous life? There are several steps we can follow to achieve this:

Choose a previous life that interests you. It can be a life that you have recently remembered or one that you have had for a long time. The important thing is that you feel attracted to it and are curious to know more about it.

Gather as much information as possible about that life. You can use the techniques we already reviewed to access more memories of that life, such as regressive hypnosis, meditation or lucid dreaming. You can also look for external sources to help you corroborate or expand the data you have, such as books, documentaries, maps, photos or testimonies of other people who have lived in that time or place. You can write down all the information you obtain in a notebook or in a digital file, organizing it by categories such as name, date, place, family, profession, important events, etc.

Analyze the information from a spiritual perspective. Once you have enough information about your previous life, you can begin to interpret it from a deeper and more transcendent point of view. You can ask yourself questions such as: What was the meaning of that life? What did I learn from it? What mistakes did I make? What karmic debts did I generate or pay off? What people did I meet and what bonds did I establish with them? What talents did I develop or waste? What fears did I overcome or reinforce? What challenges did I face or avoid? What message did that life leave me with for my present?

Apply the lessons of that life to your present life. The last step is the most important and the most difficult: integrating what you have learned from your previous life into your present life. This involves becoming aware of how that life affects you today, both positively and negatively, and making the necessary changes to improve your situation. For example, if in your previous life you were victim of an injustice, you can work to forgive those responsible and free yourself from resentment. If in your previous life you developed an artistic talent, you can take it up again or enhance it. If in your previous life you faced a great challenge, you can draw on your strength or seek to resolve it in another way.

Exploring the past is not an end in itself, but a means to better understand our present and project our future. By delving into the study of a past life, we not only discover fascinating aspects of our personal history, but also connect with our spiritual essence and life purpose. Each life is an opportunity to learn, grow and evolve as souls. By remembering our past lives, we honor our past and transform it into a gift for our present.

Guided meditation to explore in depth a specific past life.

When you are ready, close your eyes and breathe deeply. Breathe in through your nose and out through your mouth, slowly and calmly. Feel the air flow in and out of your body, filling you with energy and peace. Repeat this breathing cycle about ten times, or until you feel relaxed and calm.

Now, direct your attention to your body. Start with your feet and work your way up through your legs, knees, thighs, hips, abdomen, chest, arms, hands, shoulders, neck, face and head. Feel each part of your body and relax any tense or contracted muscles. Imagine a warm white light running through your entire body, from your feet to your head, relaxing and healing you.

Now that you are relaxed and aware of your body, let's prepare to travel back in time. Imagine that you are in a safe and beautiful place, where you feel comfortable and happy. It can be a real or imaginary place, the important thing is that it is a place that you like and that transmits peace. Visualize that place with all its details: the colors, the sounds, the smells, the sensations... Enjoy that place for a few moments and feel how it envelops you with its positive energy.

In that wonderful place, there is a door. A door that takes you to the past, to one of your previous lives. It is a special door that opens only for you and that only you can go through. Approach that door with confidence and curiosity. Observe what the door is like: its shape, its color, its material... Touch the door with your hands and feel its texture and temperature.

You are now ready to open the door and enter the past. Before you do, remember that this is a safe journey controlled by you. You decide what you want to see, what you want to feel and how long you want to stay. If at any time you feel uncomfortable or scared, you can return to the present by closing the door and opening your eyes.

When you are ready, open the door with determination and cross the threshold. In doing so, you enter another time, another life. Let your intuition guide you and observe what you see around you. Where are you? What year is it? What are you wearing? What people are with you? What are you doing?

Pay attention to all the details of that life: the place, the time, the people, the activities... Try to identify who you are in that life: your name, your age, your gender, your profession... Feel how it is to be in that life: your emotions, your thoughts, your desires...

Now that you have made contact with that previous life, let's go deeper into its study. To do this, we are going to ask some questions that will help us to better understand that life and its relationship with our current life.

What was the meaning of that life? What was the purpose of your soul in choosing that life? What did you want to learn or experience in it? Reflect for a few moments and try to find honest answers.

What did you learn in that life? What lessons did you learn from your experiences? What skills or knowledge did you acquire? What values or virtues did you develop? Think for a few moments and try to remember what you learned in that life.

What mistakes did you make in that life? What actions or decisions do you regret having made? What consequences did your mistakes have for you and for others? What karmic debts did you generate or pay off? Meditate on all this for a while and acknowledge your mistakes with humility.

What people did you meet in that life and what bonds did you establish with them? What people were important to you in that life? What role did they play in your learning? What feelings did you have towards them? What people from that life have you met again in your current life? Reflect for a few moments and thank the people who accompanied you in that life.

What message did that life leave you for your present? What advice or warning did your past self give you? What aspects of that life can you apply to your present life? What changes can you make to improve your situation? Reflect for a few moments and try to listen to your soul's message.

Now that you have deepened your study of a previous life, it is time to return to the present. Before you do, say goodbye to that life with love and gratitude. Thank your past self for all it has taught you and all it has given you. Tell it that you love it and that you forgive it. Tell it that you are proud of it and that you honor it with your current life.

Now, go back to the door that brought you to the past and carefully close it. In doing so, you return to the safe and beautiful place where you began the meditation. Feel yourself back in that place, surrounded by its positive energy. Breathe deeply and feel the air flow in and out of your lungs, filling you with vitality and joy.

When you are ready, open your eyes and come back to reality. Take a few moments to stretch, move and wake up completely. If you want, you can write down what you have seen, felt and learned in this meditation, so that you will not forget it and can refer to it later.

If you want a recorded version of this guided meditation, go to the Youtube channel of "Holos Arts Project" and search under the name: Guided meditation to explore in depth a specific past life.

You have done a great job exploring the past and delving into the study of a previous life. I hope you enjoyed this guided meditation and that it helped you to get to know yourself and your life purpose better. Remember that you can repeat this meditation whenever you want, with the same or another previous life. Each time you do it, you will discover something new and valuable about yourself and your soul.

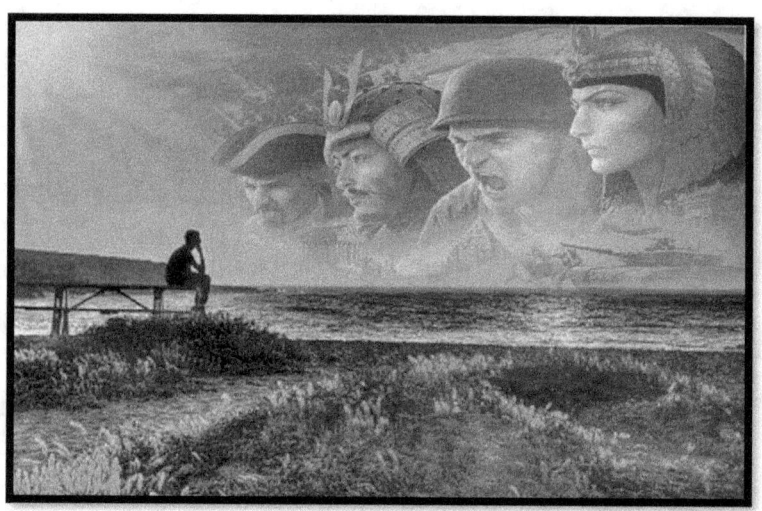

Chapter 10.

Themes and Patterns through Previous Lives

In the vast tapestry of human existence, past lives are interconnected threads that shape our present. As we delve into the fascinating world of past lives, we find ourselves with the opportunity to explore recurring themes and patterns that have left a lasting imprint on our soul. In this chapter, we will dive into the deep exploration of how to identify these themes and patterns, and how to use this knowledge for our personal growth and self-knowledge.

Discovering Common Threads

The search for recurring themes throughout past lives is like unraveling a mystery woven into the fabric of time. By looking closely at events, relationships and experiences from different eras, we begin to identify common threads that transcend the barrier of time. It may be a constant yearning for creativity, a recurring challenge in relationships, or an ongoing struggle for personal empowerment. By recognizing these themes, we dive into a deep understanding of the lessons the soul seeks to learn along its journey.

The Patterns that Weave History

Patterns are like subway rivers that run through past and present lives, influencing our choices, relationships and experiences. By carefully observing these currents, we begin to glimpse how our current actions and decisions blend into the web of patterns we have woven over time. For example, a pattern of abandonment may manifest in the way we relate to others, often repeating scenarios of loss and separation. By exploring these patterns, we provide ourselves with the opportunity to free ourselves from their limiting influence and build new ways of interacting with the world.

Working with Patterns for Personal Growth

The journey of past life discovery is not just an academic exercise, but a profound quest for self-knowledge and transformation. Once we have identified the themes and patterns, it is time to use this understanding for our personal growth. Here are some ways we can work with the patterns:

1. Mindfulness: The first step to transform a pattern is to be aware of it. By recognizing how it manifests in our lives, we gain the ability to stop its automatic repetition and make conscious decisions.

2. Deep Reflection: Taking the time to reflect on how a particular pattern has influenced our lives can help us unravel the underlying beliefs and associated emotional wounds. This allows us to heal and release the energy trapped in negative patterns.

3. Conscious Choice: By recognizing patterns, we can make conscious choices that break with the repetition of the past. Instead of following automatic reactions, we can choose responses that are aligned with our growth and well-being.

4. Therapy and Healing: The help of professionals in psychology and alternative therapies can be invaluable in addressing ingrained patterns. Techniques such as past life regression, regression therapy and energy healing can be powerful tools in this process.

5. Positive Transformation: Once we have released limiting patterns, we can replace them with new positive and empowering patterns. This involves cultivating a growth mindset and practicing new behaviors that foster our spiritual evolution.

Transformative Conclusions

In our journey of self-knowledge through past lives, we discover that we are weavers of our own destiny, influenced by threads from the past that continue to intertwine in the present. By exploring the recurring themes and patterns that have marked our soul, we open the door to healing and personal growth. This journey not only allows us to understand who we are on a deep level, but also to free ourselves from the chains of the past and transcend into a future full of possibilities.

In the next chapter, we will dive into the exciting topic of karmic connections and how interpersonal relationships reflect the bonds woven throughout past lives. Get ready for an exciting journey into understanding how souls intertwine in a cosmic dance through time.

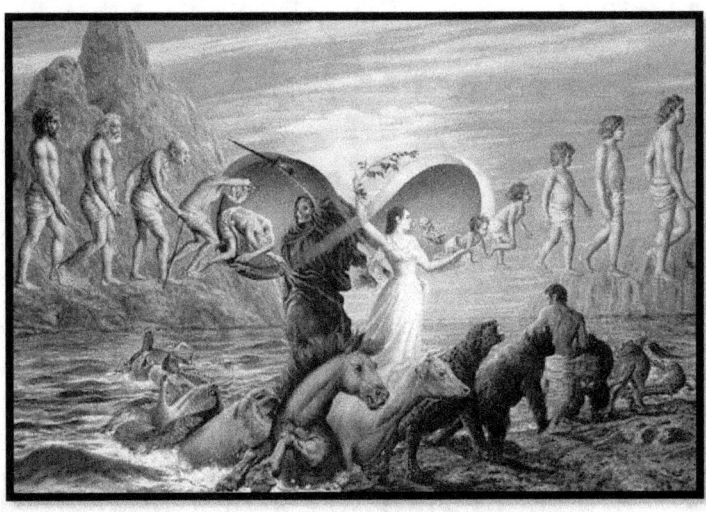

Chapter 11.

Karmic Connections:
Interpersonal Relationships Across Time

We will dive into the intriguing world of interpersonal relationships from a karmic perspective, exploring how these deep bonds influence our present lives and how we can heal and nurture these relationships for our spiritual growth.

The Bonds that Transcend Time

Karmic connections know no temporal boundaries. As we explore past lives, we begin to notice that certain people become intertwined in our memories across different times and contexts. They may be passionate loves, loyal friends or even persistent rivals. These recurring souls play a crucial role in our journey, as they embody specific lessons and challenges that our soul needs to face for its evolution.

Learning Reflections

Every karmic relationship acts as a mirror that reflects deep aspects of ourselves. It may be a quality we admire or a wound that still hurts. These connections often provoke intense reactions in us, indicating that we are touching a deep core of unfinished lessons. For example, a relationship marked by betrayal may reflect our inner struggle to trust and forgive.

Healing Through Consciousness

By exploring our karmic relationships, we open the door to the possibility of healing and transformation. Awareness is the key to releasing repetitive patterns and cycles that we have shared with these souls throughout past lives. By recognizing the lessons and unresolved emotions surrounding these relationships, we can begin to heal wounds and release the weight of the past.

Tools for Karmic Healing

1. Forgiveness and Liberation: Forgiveness is not only a gift to others, but also to ourselves. Releasing resentments and grudges allows energy to flow freely and opens space for new positive connections.

2. Deep Self-Reflection: Taking the time to reflect on the dynamics of our karmic relationships helps us to understand how they have influenced our present life. This allows us to address negative patterns and look for constructive ways to interact.

3. Authentic Communication: Talking openly and honestly with the people involved in our karmic relationships can be a powerful form of healing. Sharing our emotions and listening to those of others can open the door to understanding and reconciliation.

4. Spiritual Practices: Meditation, visualization and other spiritual practices can be effective tools for healing and nurturing our karmic relationships. Imagining a healing dialogue with the other person or sending them love and understanding can have a profound impact on our connection.

Harvesting the Fruit of Spiritual Growth

By working with our karmic connections, we are taking a bold step toward our spiritual growth. As we heal and nurture these relationships, we not only release the weight of the past, but also create space for new experiences and positive connections to flourish in our present life. We recognize that the people who come into our lives, whether to challenge or support, are allies in our evolutionary journey.

In the next chapter, we will dive into exploring how the talents and abilities we have developed over past lives manifest in our current life. Get ready to discover how the gifts of the past continue to be a source of power and potential on your path to self-realization.

Chapter 12.

Inheriting Gifts from the Past: Awakening Your Innate Talents

As we explore our past lives, it is fascinating to observe how certain talents and skills pierce the veil of time. Perhaps you were a passionate musician in the Renaissance, an intuitive healer in antiquity, or a skilled craftsman in more recent times. These gifts do not fade into the obscurity of the past; instead, they form a thread of continuity that connects your personal history in a rich narrative of evolution.

A case that exemplifies all this is that of Ismael (not his real name), a 35-year-old man who suffered from an autoimmune disease that caused pain and inflammation in his joints. Ismael had tried several medical treatments, but none gave him relief. One day, he decided to come to my office, and through my help he was able to recall a previous life in which he was a healer in an indigenous tribe. Ismael recalled that he had the gift of healing people with his hands and with medicinal plants, and that he was highly respected by his community. He also remembered that he died young, the victim of an ambush by another rival group.

I explained to Ismael that his current illness was the result of a conflict between his soul and his body, because in this life he had forgotten his purpose and his mission to heal. I suggested that he reconnect with his ancestral wisdom and practice self-healing with his hands, visualizing the energy flowing through his body and healing him. I also recommended that he research the medicinal plants he used in his past life and incorporate them into his diet and routine.

Ismael followed my advice and began to notice an improvement in his health. He felt calmer, more confident and happier. He discovered that some of the plants he used in his past life were aloe, ginger and turmeric, and that they had anti-inflammatory and antioxidant properties. He also learned to use his hands to channel energy and relieve pain, following the principles of reiki. Eventually, Ismael was completely cured of his illness, and dedicated himself to helping others with his healing knowledge.

Recognizing the Gifts of the Past

The first step in awakening your past gifts is to recognize them. Often, these talents manifest as deep interests, natural inclinations, or skills that develop easily. Reflect on what you love to do and how you feel most alive. Do you have an innate affinity for the visual arts, an ability to understand complex patterns, or a gift for connecting with the emotions of others? These could be traces of gifts rooted in previous lives.

Leveraging the Gifts in the Present

Awakening and tapping into your past gifts is an act of empowerment and self-discovery. Here are some ways you can cultivate and nurture your innate abilities:

1. Education and Practice: If you feel a pull toward a particular field, look for opportunities to learn and practice. Taking classes, attending workshops or immersing yourself in study helps you refine your skills and develop your full potential.

2. Creative Integration: If you have an artistic or creative talent, look for ways to incorporate these expressions into your daily life. It can be painting, writing, dancing or any other activity that allows you to channel your creativity.

3. Share with others: Sharing your gifts with others not only enriches their lives, but also gives you an opportunity for personal growth. You can teach, offer your help or simply show your art or skills to the world.

4. Meditation and Inner Exploration: Meditation and introspection can help you connect with your past lives and consciously access the gifts you carry with you. Visualize how you used your abilities in previous lives and how you can apply them in your current life.

A Celebration of Evolution

As you awaken and nurture your past gifts, you are participating in a celebration of your spiritual evolution. You recognize that you are an embodiment of skills and talents accumulated over time, and that each past experience has contributed to who you are today. By tapping into these gifts, you not only enrich your own life, but you also contribute to the beauty and enrichment of the world around you.

Chapter 13.

Exploring Diverse Lives and Past Cultures

On the vast horizon of our past lives, cultural and social landscapes unfold as diverse as the stars in the sky. In this chapter, we venture on an exciting journey through lives in different times and places, exploring the profound lessons we can learn from ancient cultures and societies. As we unravel the threads of history, we discover how those experiences enrich our present lives and connect us to the rich diversity of human experience.

Crossing Temporary Borders

The exploration of past lives allows us to cross the boundaries of time and immerse ourselves in remote times and places. We can walk the streets of ancient Roman cities, contemplate the splendor of Egyptian civilizations or feel the earth beneath our feet in a medieval village. Through this experience, we broaden our perspective and connect with the deep roots of humanity.

Learning from Ancient Cultures and Societies

Each culture and society has its own unique set of values, beliefs and challenges. By exploring past lives in different cultural contexts, we have the opportunity to tap into worlds of knowledge and wisdom that can enrich our current understanding. We can learn from the life philosophies of the ancient Greeks, the connection to nature of indigenous peoples or the deep spirituality of Eastern traditions.

Universal Lessons Through Time

Despite cultural and temporal differences, there are universal lessons that transcend the ages and remain guiding lights for human growth. Love, compassion, perseverance and the search for meaning are examples of core values that have manifested throughout human history. By exploring past lives, we discover how these lessons are woven into the individual and collective experiences of different eras.

Reflections on the Present

The exploration of past lives in diverse cultures and societies invites us to reflect on how those experiences impact us in the present. Here are some considerations to enrich our current understanding:

1. Deep Connection: As we discover past lives in different cultural contexts, we develop a deeper connection to human diversity and learn to appreciate the richness of experience in all its forms.

2. Transcendental Wisdom: The teachings and wisdom of ancient cultures can offer us unique perspectives on life and purpose. We can apply these lessons to our own path of spiritual growth.

3. Resilience and Adaptability: By exploring past lives in times of change and challenge, we recognize the innate human capacity to adapt and overcome obstacles. These lessons can inspire us to face our own challenges with resilience.

4. Growth and Evolution: The variety of roles and experiences we have had in different cultures and societies shows us the versatility of our soul and our ability to grow and evolve over time.

A Mosaic of Human Experiences

Each past life is like a unique piece of an intricate mosaic that represents the human experience throughout the ages. As we explore lives in different times and places, we weave a tapestry in which our own stories are interwoven with the stories of humanity. In this union of past and present, we find inspiration to embrace our own uniqueness and contribute to the ongoing enrichment of the larger story of humanity.

Chapter 14.

Anne's Journey: A Mosaic of Past Lives

Ana (not her real name), a thirty-five-year-old woman, came to my office in search of profound answers and a greater understanding of herself. She had experienced unexplainable feelings and emotions throughout her life and felt an intense connection to certain cultures and places that she could not explain. We decided to explore her experience through past life regression therapy in an effort to shed light on her situation.

During her first regression, Ana was gently guided into a state of deep relaxation. As she began to deepen her awareness, she found herself in an entirely different time and place: she was a brave warrior in ancient Rome. She experienced the intensity of battle and the camaraderie among fellow soldiers. However, in later sessions, and as we continued to explore other incarnations, Ana also experienced past lives as a woman, embodying roles ranging from a shaman in a Native American tribe to a nun in medieval Europe.

What transpired was that Ana had not only experienced past lives in different times and countries but had also occupied both male and female bodies. This variety of gender experiences presented itself seamlessly and naturally on her regression journey.

What is common in our spiritual journey through incarnations is that we live the whole existential spectrum: we change gender, country, culture, race and situation. Our soul needs all these experiences in order to learn what it means to come to this earthly plane and to be human.

Universal Lessons and Personal Growth

As we explored each of Ana's past lives, recurring patterns and themes emerged. Despite superficial differences in gender, culture and context, it became clear that Ana had been learning universal lessons throughout her incarnations. Courage, compassion, love and the search for meaning were values that resonated throughout her past lives, regardless of time and place.

Ana's experience reminds us of the richness of the human experience and how our souls can embody a variety of identities and roles in search of growth and evolution. Ana was able to see how her previous experiences had influenced her current personality and challenges, and how the lessons learned throughout her past lives could be applied to her quest for self-discovery and self-realization in the present.

Integration and Healing

Past life regression provided Ana with a unique and enlightening perspective on her own spiritual history. It allowed her to understand her deep interaction with different cultures and places, as well as the fluidity of her gender identity over time.

Ana used this understanding to heal emotional wounds and release limiting patterns that had persisted throughout their lives.

Chapter 15.

The Importance of Forgiveness and Self-Compassion in the study of past lives.

As we explore past lives, it is inevitable that we will encounter moments of pain, betrayal and loss. These wounds may have been caused by our own actions or by the actions of others toward us. However, regardless of the source, these wounds can creep through time and affect our present life in subtle or overt ways. Often, these chains from the past prevent us from moving forward and experiencing the fulfillment we long for.

The Power of Forgiveness

Forgiveness is a golden key that can free us from the clutches of the past. By forgiving others and ourselves for past hurts and offenses, we release a healing energy that transcends temporal barriers. Forgiving does not mean justifying negative actions, but freeing ourselves from the emotional weight we carry. As we explore past lives and encounter situations that require forgiveness, let us remember that forgiveness is a gift we give ourselves.

Healing Through Self-Love

Self-compassion is an essential component of healing through past lives. Some of the wounds we encounter may be the result of our own actions or decisions in previous lives. Cultivating self-compassion allows us to recognize that, as human beings, we are fallible and in a constant process of learning. We give ourselves permission to accept our imperfections and learn from them without harshly judging ourselves.

The Cycle of Growth and Healing

When we practice forgiveness and self-compassion in the context of past lives, we are participating in a profound cycle of growth and healing. By releasing past hurts and guilt, we create space for transformation and flourishing. Lessons learned from past lives become powerful tools to guide our present choices and actions in a wiser and more loving way.

The Final Release

Past life exploration provides us with the opportunity to experience a final and profound release. As we forgive and practice self-compassion, we release the emotional attachments that have kept us entangled in repetitive cycles. We open ourselves to the possibility of living with greater authenticity and joy in the present, honoring our spiritual history without being trapped in it.

In our journey through past lives, forgiveness and self-compassion reveal themselves as precious gems on the path of healing and spiritual growth. By practicing these qualities, we honor our self in all its incarnations and create a solid foundation for wholeness and liberation. As we bring these lessons into our daily lives, we weave a tapestry of love and understanding that transcends time and space, guiding us toward a state of inner peace and fulfillment.

Chapter 16.

Exploring Future Lives:
A Glimpse of What Can Be

So far, our journey has been through the lens of the past, revealing the hidden gems of previous lives. However, the spiritual journey is not limited to the history that has already been written. In this chapter, we will venture beyond the boundaries of time and explore the intriguing possibility of future lives. Through this exploration, we will get a glimpse of what might be waiting for us beyond the time horizon, and how we can harness this knowledge to shape our present and future.

The Future as a Possibility

The idea of exploring future lives may seem like a mysterious and challenging concept. Time, as we perceive it, is a linear dimension, but in the spiritual realm, temporal limitations are blurred. Instead of seeing the future as an immutable certainty, we can understand it as a series of possibilities that unfold based on our present choices and actions.

The Journey of Intuition and Imagination

The exploration of future lives is often done through intuition and imagination. Through meditation, hypnosis and visualization techniques, we can connect with our soul's future potential. Imagine being in an unfamiliar environment, taking on roles and experiences that could be part of our next incarnation. Through this journey, we can access deep insights and knowledge that reside within our being.

Continuing Lessons and Future Purpose

In exploring future lives, we may also find recurring patterns and themes that reflect ongoing lessons and purposes in our spiritual evolution. If in our past lives we have been working on compassion, self-reliance or authenticity, it is likely that these lessons will continue to be relevant in our future lives. This exploration can offer us greater clarity about where we should focus in our quest for growth and self-realization.

The Wisdom of Conscious Choices

Although the future is fluid and full of possibilities, our exploration of future lives can offer us a window into what could be if we follow certain directions. By understanding how our present choices can influence our future lives, we gain a greater sense of responsibility and empowerment over our spiritual evolution. This encourages us to make conscious choices that are aligned with our true essence.

Living the Present with Consciousness

The exploration of future lives is not intended to distract us from the present, but to enrich our understanding of how our current choices and actions have a long-term impact. By living with full awareness and considering the lessons learned from past lives and the possibilities of future lives, we create a state of balance and harmony in which we are more connected to our true essence.

Future life exploration invites us to embrace the uncertainty of the future with empowerment and curiosity. Through this exploration, we understand that we are the creators of our own reality, able to shape our destiny through conscious choices aligned with our spiritual purpose. As we continue our journey in this life and beyond, we carry with us the wisdom of our past lives and the possibilities of future lives, weaving a unique tapestry of experience and growth on the vast canvas of time.

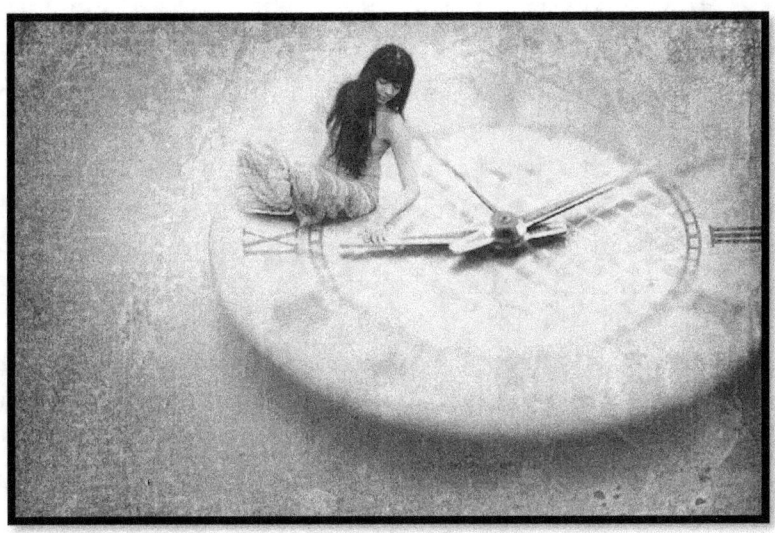

Chapter 17.

Guided Meditation:
Exploring Your Future Life

Before beginning this meditation, make sure you are in a quiet, comfortable place where you will not be interrupted. Sit or lie down in a relaxed position, close your eyes and take a few deep breaths to enter a state of deep relaxation. Imagine each inhalation filling you with positive energy and each exhalation releasing any tension or worries.

Visualize that you are surrounded by a warm, white light, creating a protective and loving shield around you. Feel how this light fills you with calm and serenity, allowing you to enter a space of deep introspection and spiritual connection.

Imagine that you are climbing a gentle hill covered with green grass. As you go, you feel a loving and wise presence by your side, this is your spiritual guide. Feel its calming energy and limitless wisdom as it leads you on this journey of exploration.

You reach the top of the hill and before you stands an ancient carved wooden door. This door represents the threshold to your future life. You feel the texture of the wood under your hands and the anticipation in the air as you prepare to walk through it. You know that this door will lead you to a vision of possible future moments.

With determination and curiosity, you open the door and cross the threshold into an ever-changing landscape. You find yourself in a place that is both familiar and strange. Observe the details around you: the light, the colors, the sounds. Take a moment to absorb the atmosphere and tune into the energy of the future.

You continue to walk through this environment, exploring the places and people you encounter. As you move forward, you become aware of the presence of someone in the distance. As you get closer, you realize that it is a future version of yourself. Observe carefully how this version of you is doing in your future life: your appearance, your activities, your surroundings.

Feel free to approach your future self and engage him or her in conversation. You can ask questions about his or her life, his or her experiences and the lessons he or she has learned. Listen carefully to his or her words and observe the emotions that arise within you as you interact with this version of yourself.

Now, ask your future self to reveal to you any important lessons or purposes that you need to carry out in your present life. What is the best advice your future self can give your present self? Pay attention to the words and images that arise in your mind. These revelations can help you better understand your path and your spiritual growth.

When you are ready to conclude this exploration, thank your future self for sharing its wisdom with you. Visualize the wooden door once again and feel ready to cross back to the present. As you close the door, carry with you the lessons and positive energy you have found in your future life.

Slowly begin to bring your awareness back to your current environment. Feel the connection to the space around you and begin to gently wiggle your fingers and toes. When you feel ready, open your eyes and take a moment to take in the experience.

Take note of the impressions, emotions and lessons that emerged during this guided meditation. Reflect on how you can apply this wisdom in your present life. Remember that the future is not set in stone and that your current choices and actions can influence the possibilities that lie ahead.

Allow yourself to return to this meditation whenever you wish to explore your future life and gain guidance on your present spiritual path. With each exploration, you are weaving a deeper link between your past, your present and the limitless possibilities of your future.

For a recorded version of this meditation, go to the Holos Arts Project Youtube Channel and search for the video: Guided Meditation, Exploring Your Future Life.

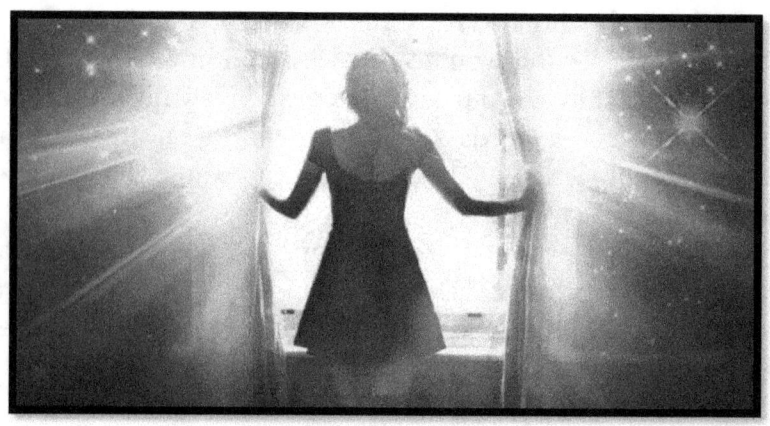

Chapter 18.

My personal experience during the exploration of the period between lives

The period between lives is the time that elapses between one incarnation and another, that is, between one physical life and another. During this period, the soul is in a spiritual plane, where it can rest, meet other like-minded souls, review its past life, learn from its mistakes and successes, plan its next life and prepare to be reborn.

The spiritual plane between lives is a place of light, love and wisdom, where the soul can access a broader and deeper vision of its reality. There, the soul can count on the help of spiritual guides and masters, who are more evolved souls that offer guidance and support. It can also access the akashic library, which is the record of all the information and memory of the universe, where it can find the answers to its existential questions.

The period between lives is an opportunity for the growth and evolution of the soul, as it allows it to become aware of its purpose, karma and destiny. The soul freely chooses the conditions of its next life, according to what it wants to experience and learn. The soul also chooses the people it will relate to in its next life, according to the affective or karmic links it has with them.

The period between lives has no fixed duration but depends on each soul and its needs. Some souls may remain on the spiritual plane between lifetimes for centuries, while others may reincarnate quickly. The period between lives may also vary according to the historical epoch and the level of collective consciousness.

The period between lives is a fascinating and mysterious subject, which has been studied by different religious, philosophical and scientific traditions. Some ways to access the memory of this period are regressive hypnosis, meditation or intuition.

Relating my personal experience

During a self-hypnosis regression, I had a transcendental experience that left me reflecting for many weeks, and also motivated me to continue preparing and studying to become a past life therapist. I was only 20 years old, but the experience definitely moved me and pushed me to follow the path of supporting other people to know their past lives. Below, I will give a rough account of what I experienced during that regression:

After recalling some of my past lives, I became very curious about what happened between lives. Where did my soul go when I left my physical body? What did I do there? Who did I meet? What did I learn? I wanted to explore the spiritual plane between lives, that mysterious and wonderful place where souls rest, reunite and prepare for their next incarnation.

To access this plane, I needed to enter a state of deep relaxation and self-hypnosis. I lay down on my bed, closed my eyes and breathed deeply. I focused on my heart, in the center of my chest, where I felt a warm, loving light. I imagined that light spreading throughout my body, filling me with peace and harmony. Then, I imagined that light rising above my body, taking me with it. I felt myself detach from my physical body and soar into the sky.

As I ascended, I saw the world from a different perspective. I saw the houses, the trees, the rivers, the mountains, the clouds... Everything looked smaller and farther away. I felt a sense of freedom and joy. I continued to climb until I reached a point where I could see nothing but a bright white light. I stepped into that light and felt enveloped by it.

The light was soft and cozy. I felt at home. It was as if I was back where I came from, where I belonged. I felt surrounded by love and understanding. I heard a sweet, familiar voice saying to me:

- Welcome back, dear friend. We are very happy to see you.

I opened my eyes and saw in front of me a luminous and beautiful being. It was one of my spiritual guides, a wise and loving soul who had accompanied me in many of my lives. I recognized him instantly and felt a great emotion. I hugged him with gratitude and told him:

- Thank you for being here, dear guide. I am also very happy to see you. I still have a lot to learn.
- I know. That's why we're here, to help you learn and grow.

My guide took me by the hand and led me to a wonderful place. It was like a garden full of flowers, trees, fountains, animals... Everything was harmonious. There I met other luminous and beautiful beings. They were my other spiritual guides, accompanied by my kindred souls. They were souls with whom I had a special connection, with whom I had shared many experiences in different lives. Some were family, friends, partners... While others were unknown to me in this life, but I recognized them by the affinity I felt with them.

Everyone received me with love and joy. They hugged me, kissed me, congratulated me... I felt very loved and valued. I felt part of a great spiritual family.

My main guide told me:

- Isis, we have come to this place to share with you our wisdom and our experience. We want to help you

understand your soul's purpose, the meaning of your past lives and the plan for your present life.
- Thank you, dear guide. I am very interested to know all that.
- We know. That's why we brought you here.

My main guide led me to a special place inside the garden. It was like a giant library filled with ancient and sacred books. Each book contained the story of a life, of a soul, of a world. My guide said to me:

- This is the akashic library, the record of all information and memory of the universe. Here you can find the answer to any question you have about your past, your present or your future.
- Can I read any of these books?
- You can read the book you request. You only have to ask for it with a very definite intention and the book will come to you.
- And how do I know which book to order?
- Well, it depends on what you want to know. You can ask for the book of your soul, the book of your current life, the book of one of your past lives, the book of your next life, the book of a subject that interests you...
- And what if I ask for the book of my next life? Isn't that supposed to be a mystery?
- It is not a mystery. It is a choice. You choose your next life before you are born. You choose the circumstances, the people, the lessons, the challenges... You choose what you want to experience and learn in each life.
- And why do we choose that? Wouldn't it be easier to choose a happy and peaceful life?
- No, Isis. It's not about being happy or peaceful. It's about being conscious and evolving. Every life is an

opportunity to grow and to express your true essence. Every life is a school where you learn what you need to learn to advance on your spiritual path.

- And how do we know what we need to learn?

- We know this because of our karma. Karma is the law of cause and effect that governs our evolution. Karma is the result of our actions, thoughts and emotions in each lifetime. Karma is what causes us to be born again and again until we learn what we need to learn.

- And what do we have to learn?

- We have to learn to love, Isis. To love ourselves, to love others, to love life, to love God. Love is the most powerful force in the universe. Love is what creates us, sustains us and unites us. Love is our nature and our destiny.

- And how do we learn to love?

- We learn to love through free will, Isis. Free will is the ability to choose between good and evil, between light and darkness, between love and fear. Free will is what makes us responsible for our lives and our souls. Free will is what makes us human.

- What if we choose wrong, what if we choose evil, darkness or fear?

- For we suffer the consequences, Isis. We suffer the pain, the guilt, the regret... We suffer the lessons we have not learned. We suffer the karma we have generated.

- And how can we free ourselves from karma?

- We can free ourselves from karma through forgiveness, Isis. Forgiveness is the ability to let go of the past, to accept the present and to trust in the future. Forgiveness is the ability to heal our wounds, to reconcile with ourselves and others. Forgiveness is the capacity to transform our karma into grace.

- And what is grace?
- Grace is the divine blessing, Isis. Grace is the unconditional help we receive from God and our spiritual guides. Grace is the light that illuminates our path and guides us to our destiny.
- And what is our destiny?
- Our destiny is enlightenment, Isis. Enlightenment is the state of fulfillment and happiness that we attain when we free ourselves from the cycle of reincarnation. Enlightenment is the state of unity and harmony with all that exists. Enlightenment is the state of pure and unconditional love.

My guide looked at me with a smile and said:

- Isis, you have asked many questions and received many answers. But remember that words are not enough to understand the truth. Truth is lived, felt, experienced. That is why we invite you to explore the spiritual plane between lives for yourself. Here you can find everything you seek and more. Here you can see your soul, your essence, your light. Here you can see the soul of others, their essence, their light. Here you can see God's soul, his essence, his light.
- How can I do that, dear guide?
- You just have to follow your heart, Isis. Your heart is your compass, your guide, your connection. Your heart knows where to go, what to do, what to say. Your heart is the organ of love.
- What if I get lost, dear guide?
- Don't worry, Isis. You can't get lost. We are with you at all times. We are here to support, protect and guide you. We are here to love you.
- Thank you, dear guide. You are very kind and generous.

My guide let go of my hand and gave me a hug. Then he said to me:

- We wish you the best in your adventure. Remember that you can always come back to this place whenever you want. We will be waiting for you here with open arms.
- Thank you, dear guide. I thank you for all you have done for me.

My guide walked away and left me alone in the akashic library. I felt a mixture of excitement and nervousness. I didn't know what I would find there, but I was ready to find out.

I approached one of the shelves and asked with my sincere intention for the book about the future of my current life. Instantly, a book appeared in my hands. It was a thick, heavy book, with a dark blue cover and gold lettering that read, "Current Life of Isis."

I opened and read the book carefully and noticed that as of the present moment it was filled only with blank pages. I was surprised and wondered if there was something wrong with the book or with me.

Then I heard a voice in my mind telling me:

- There is nothing wrong with the book or with you. The book is empty because your life is not yet written. You are the author of your own story. You are the creator of your own reality.
- What do you mean by that?
- I mean that you have the power to choose how your life will be. You have the power to decide what you want to experience and learn in it. You have the power to write your destiny. All human beings have the power to write theirs.

- And how can I do that?
- You can do it using your imagination, Isis. Your imagination is the most powerful tool you have to create your reality. Your imagination is the expression of your soul.
- And what do I have to imagine?
- Whatever makes you happy, whatever makes you grow, whatever makes you love.
- And how do I know if I'm imagining right?
- You can tell by how you feel. If you feel good, you're imagining good. If you feel bad, you're imagining bad.
- What if I imagine something bad?
- You attract it into your life. What you imagine comes true.
- What if I imagine something good?
- Well, you attract it into your life too, Isis. What you imagine comes true.
- So I can imagine anything I want and it will come true?
- Yes, this is how the law of attraction works.
- What is the law of attraction?
- It is the law that governs creation. It is the law that says like attracts like. It is the law that says that your thoughts, emotions and actions determine your reality.
- And how can I use this law to my advantage?
- You can use it to your advantage by being aware of what you think, feel and do. You can use it to your advantage by being positive, optimistic and grateful. You can use it to your advantage by being loving, compassionate and generous.
- And that will help me create a good life?
- Yes, Isis. That will help you create a wonderful life.
- What if I don't?
- You will harm yourself. You will create a difficult life for yourself.

- And why would I do that?
- Because you don't love yourself enough. Because you don't value yourself enough. Because you don't respect yourself enough.
- And how can I change that?
- You can change it by loving yourself more, Isis. You can change it by valuing yourself more. You can change it by respecting yourself more.
- And how can I do that?
- You can do this by recognizing your divinity. You can do it by recognizing that you are a child of God, like all human beings. You can do it by recognizing that human beings are beings of light.

The voice quieted and left me in thought. I realized that I had a lot to learn about myself and about the spiritual plane.

I looked at the book in my hands and felt a spark of inspiration. I decided to start writing my own story.

I took a pencil and wrote on the first page:

"In this life I want to be..."

Chapter 19.

Healing at the Collective Level

In a world that constantly seeks healing and transformation, an understanding of our past lives has emerged as a beacon of light in the darkness. The idea that our past experiences influence our present lives is not new, but in recent times, this notion has taken a profound and significant turn. Healing through past lives on a collective and global level has become a journey towards reconciliation and healing on a scale that encompasses all of humanity.

Imagine past lives as the pages of a cosmic book containing the history of humanity. On each page, there are events, emotions and decisions that have left an imprint on the collective soul. These imprints, often called "karmic wounds," can influence our behavior, relationships and thought patterns in this lifetime. Healing through past lives thus becomes an exploration of these wounds and the release of trapped energies that still affect humanity.

On a broader level, our past lives are intertwined in an intricate web of connections. Events that occurred in times past can have resonances in the present. For example, historical conflicts and collective traumas can manifest in the form of social tensions, inequalities and prejudices in the present. By healing these wounds in the present through the exploration and healing of previous incarnations, we are contributing to the healing of the larger fabric of human history.

Group healing practices and meditations are like gemstones that reflect the light of the collective consciousness. By coming together in groups with similar intentions, we create an energy field that is far more powerful than the sum of its individual parts. Group healing sessions can focus on specific issues, such as healing historical traumas, reconciliation between groups, or releasing destructive patterns rooted in the past.

Group meditations are gateways to the transpersonal dimension, where the limitations of time and space fade away. In this space, we can connect with ancient wisdom, spirit guides and beings of light who assist us in the healing process on a collective level. Meditation allows us to enter into deep communion with kindred souls from around the world, creating a unified field of intention and healing.

Each individual, by consciously exploring his or her past lives, has the potential to become an agent of change in the collective fabric of humanity. Past life exploration invites us to look beyond the boundaries of this life and recognize that we are eternal beings who have experienced countless incarnations. This broader perspective allows us to transcend superficial divisions and embrace the deep connection we share with all souls.

As we explore our past lives, it is essential to approach this process with an open heart and a spirit of curiosity. The memories that emerge may be poignant, shocking or surprising. Some may lead us to confront old conflicts or unresolved challenges that still resonate in the present. Healing occurs when we face these experiences with compassion and empathy, releasing the power they hold over us.

By releasing limiting patterns and healing wounds on a personal level, we create a cascading effect that ripples through time and space. Our actions, thoughts and emotions reverberate in the collective consciousness, influencing the way humanity relates to itself and the world around it. In this sense, each individual becomes a beacon of light that illuminates the darkness and guides others toward healing and transformation.

Healing through past lives on a collective and global level is a journey in which each individual has a vital role to play. As we explore our past lives, we release the chains of the past and allow healing to flow through time. Group healing practices and meditations amplify this process, creating energy fields that transcend the barriers of time and space. By healing ourselves, we contribute to the well-being of humanity as a whole, we weave threads of love and understanding into the tapestry of reality and pave the way for a brighter, more unified future.

Chapter 20.

Integrating the Consciousness of the Immortality of the Soul

An eternal truth awaits our perception and acceptance: the immortality of the soul. As we expand our consciousness to embrace this perspective, our ingrained concepts of life and death are transformed into a cosmic dance of understanding and transcendence. In this chapter, we will explore how awareness of the immortality of the soul can revolutionize our perception of existence, how this new vision invites us to live fully in the present, and how transcending time allows us to experience an enriched and meaningful life.

Embracing the prospect of the immortality of the soul

Since time immemorial, cultures and philosophies around the world have hinted at the idea that the soul is eternal and transcends earthly experience. However, in modern society, this notion has often been relegated to the dark corners of spirituality, overshadowed by a materialistic mindset that emphasizes tangible, observable reality. However, the awakening of individual consciousness is bringing with it a resurgence of this ancient wisdom, challenging the limitations imposed by the rational mind and opening the doors to a deeper perception of reality.

The immortality of the soul does not simply refer to a perpetual existence after physical death, but to the idea that our essence transcends the limitations of time and form. This understanding challenges our linear perception of time and invites us to consider that our souls exist beyond the conventional conception of past, present and future. By embracing this perspective, we free ourselves from the shackles of mortality and immerse ourselves in an ocean of infinite possibilities.

How this consciousness transforms our perception of life and death.

Awareness of the immortality of the soul opens a portal to a new understanding of life and death. Death, once considered an abrupt and dreaded end, becomes a transit to another phase of existence. Understanding that our essence is indestructible and that our history is much broader than the present life, we experience a profound change in the way we face the inevitability of death.

Life takes on a deeper nuance when we realize that our present experiences are only a small part of an eternal journey. Every challenge, joy and encounter takes on a broader meaning in the context of our immortal existence. Instead of anxiously clinging to fleeting pleasures or lamenting momentary difficulties, we adopt a more serene and balanced perspective that values the experience itself and the learning it brings to our eternal being.

Living fully in the present knowing that our existence transcends time.

When we understand that our existence spans multiple incarnations and transcends linear time, our relationship to the present is transformed. Instead of obsessively focusing on the accumulation of material possessions or the constant pursuit of external achievements, we turn inward and find meaning in the journey itself. Each moment becomes an opportunity to explore, grow and connect more deeply with our true essence.

Awareness of the immortality of the soul enables us to free ourselves from the trivial worries and superficial anxieties that often ensnare us. While we still face challenges and obstacles along the way, we are able to face them with renewed peace of mind and purpose. We know that we are more than our present circumstances and that each experience contributes to our spiritual growth and evolution throughout the ages.

Living fully in the present also involves a deep appreciation for the interconnectedness of all things. We recognize that every action we take, every thought we generate and every emotion we experience reverberates through time and space. Our influence transcends the boundaries of the individual and extends into the very fabric of the universe.

The integration of the awareness of the immortality of the soul is a journey of profound self-discovery and expansion of perception. As we embrace the idea that our souls are eternal and transcend time, we experience a radical transformation in the way we view life and death. Our perspective expands beyond temporal limitations and allows us to live fully in the present, knowing that our current experiences are only a small part of an ever-evolving cosmic journey.

The immortality of the soul invites us to explore the vastness of our own essence and to understand that we are eternal beings in search of self-transcendence. By embracing this understanding, we find profound peace in the certainty that our souls are unshakable and that our existence has a transcendent purpose that goes beyond earthly limitations. Ultimately, the integration of this awareness guides us into a life of greater wisdom, connection and meaning, as we rise above the veil of time and step into the infinite vastness of existence.

Chapter 21.

Conclusions, Embracing the Weaving of Our Past Stories

Dear readers, it has been an amazing and revealing journey that we have undertaken together through these pages. We have explored the deepest corners of our being, unraveling the mysteries of our past lives and discovering the invisible threads that connect our personal history to the larger fabric of humanity. At the end of this book, I invite you to pause for a moment and reflect on the journey you have undertaken and the doors you have opened toward understanding yourself and the story you carry within.

Exploring our past incarnations is an act of courage and self-discovery. Throughout these pages, we have explored how our past lives can influence our current experiences and challenges, how recurring patterns can be rooted in unresolved past experiences, and how healing in the present can have a profound and transformative impact on all dimensions of our being. But this exploration goes beyond the words printed in these pages; it is an intimate and personal journey that will continue to resonate in your heart and mind long after you have closed this book.

You may have been surprised to discover deep connections to people and places you had never known before. Perhaps you have experienced moments of clarity and understanding, as if a light has been shed on the unknowns of your life. Or you may have felt overwhelming and liberating emotions as you faced past traumas and allowed healing to flow through your being. Whatever your experience, I want you to know that you have taken a courageous step toward your own growth and transformation.

The journey of discovering your past lives is an invitation to explore the deepest layers of your being and to unearth the hidden gems of ancient wisdom that reside within you. Each incarnation you have explored is like a piece of the puzzle of your existence, and by putting these pieces together, you are creating a more complete and enriching picture of who you really are. As you delve deeper into the depths of your being, you get closer to the truth of your eternal self and discover the lessons and purposes that have guided your incarnations over the centuries.

As you look back on this journey, remember that the answers you have found are only the beginning. The past lives you have explored are like doors that open to vast expanses of knowledge and understanding. Continue to walk these corridors of time with curiosity and longing, knowing that each step brings you closer to the profound truth that resides deep within you.

If this exploration of past lives has awakened your interest in alternative therapies and the deeper dimensions of consciousness, I invite you to continue your search. This book is just a starting point, a spark that ignites the flame of exploration and transformation. I encourage you to explore my other books that address topics related to holistic healing, spirituality and personal growth. Each book is a window into new perspectives and opportunities to expand your understanding and experience of life.

If you wish to receive your diploma of completion, please write to the following email: holosartsproject@gmail.com

As you close this book and continue your journey, I want you to know that you are on a path of self-discovery that knows no bounds. You are a spark of consciousness in the vast universe, and your past life explorations are like constellations of stars that light your path. Allow yourself to continue to be guided by that inner light, allowing it to take you to new depths of understanding.

From the bottom of my heart, I want to thank you for joining me on this journey. It is an honor to have shared these pages with you. May you continue to explore, grow and heal as you embrace the wondrous and eternal dance of existence. Until our paths cross again, I send you love, gratitude and sincere wishes for peace and fulfillment in all your future journeys.

With love and gratitude,
Isis Estrada.

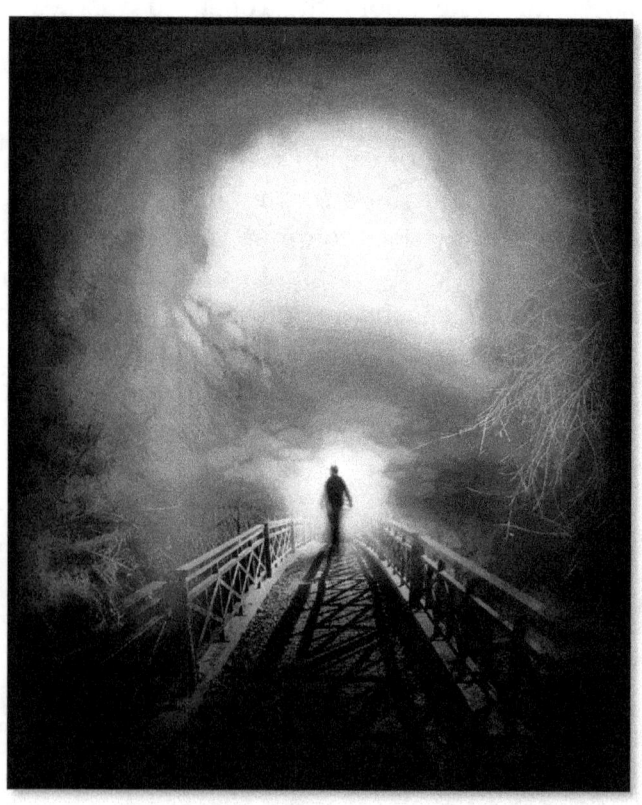

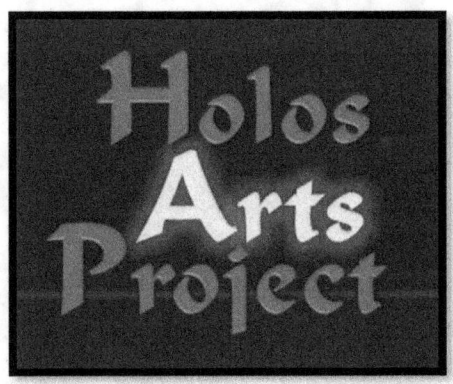

We at Holos Arts Project are grateful for your reading this book. If the content has left you satisfied, you can give us a rating on the Amazon website. We invite you to keep in touch with us, through our website to be aware of the latest news.

https://www.holosartsproject.com
https://centrodeterapiasalternativas.weebly.com/

Social Networks
Facebook, official profile: Holos Arts
Facebook, official page: Holos Arts Project
Instagram: HolosArts and CentroSenderoMístico
Youtube: Holos Arts Project
E-mail: holosartsproject@gmail.com

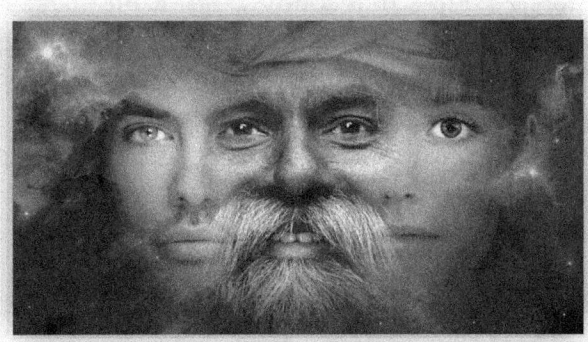

OTHER BOOKS BY ISIS ESTRADA

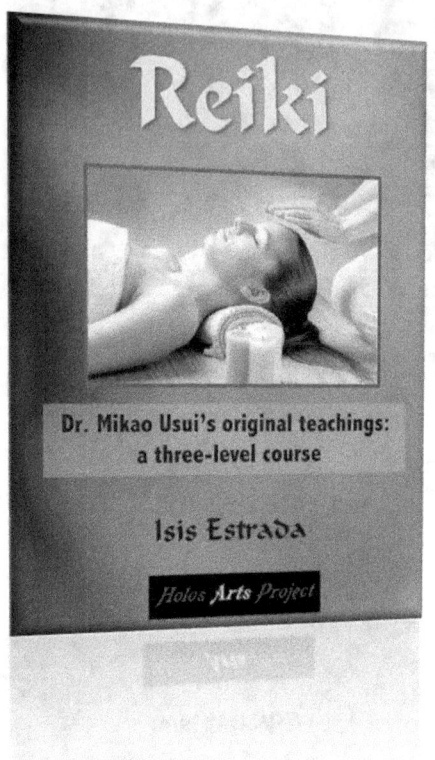

**Reiki: Dr. Mikao Usui's original teachings,
a three-level course.**

Complete course that follows the traditional teachings of Dr. Mikao Usui, discoverer of the use of universal energy for healing. The psychologist Isis Estrada, has compiled this manual as a complete course, which includes the attunements and the information of all the Reiki wisdom, beginner, practitioner and master levels.
Buy it on Amazon, in print or digital versions.

https://www.amazon.com/Reiki-original-teachings-three-level-course/dp/B0C9SK1RGR/

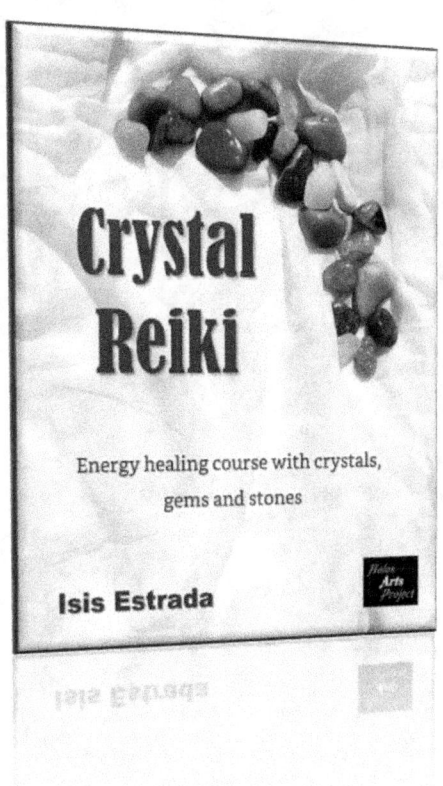

Crystal Reiki:
Energy healing course with crystals, gems and stones

A book that progresses from the basics to advanced techniques in the application of the properties of crystals in Reiki healing sessions. The book includes the attunement as well as an accredited Reiki master diploma.

https://www.amazon.com/Crystal-Reiki-Energy-healing-crystals/dp/B0CCCSTPDV

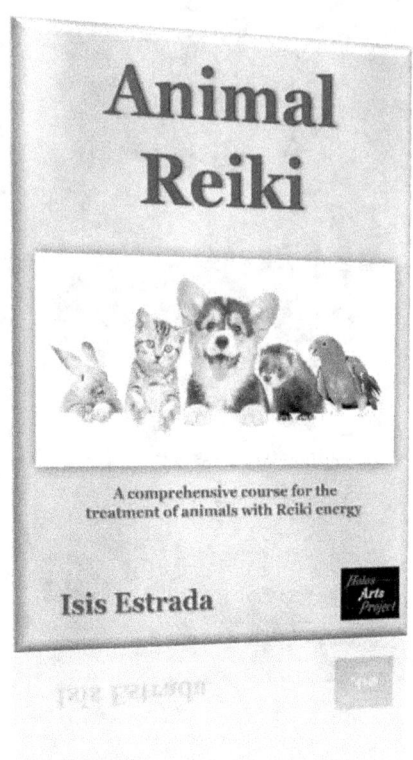

Animal Reiki: A complete Course for the Treatment of Animals with Reiki energy

A book dedicated to learn the technique to keep our pets healthy with the universal energy of Reiki. The book includes the attunement, as well as an accredited Reiki master diploma.
https://www.amazon.com/Animal-Reiki-comprehensive-treatment-animals/dp/B0CCXHY1NK/

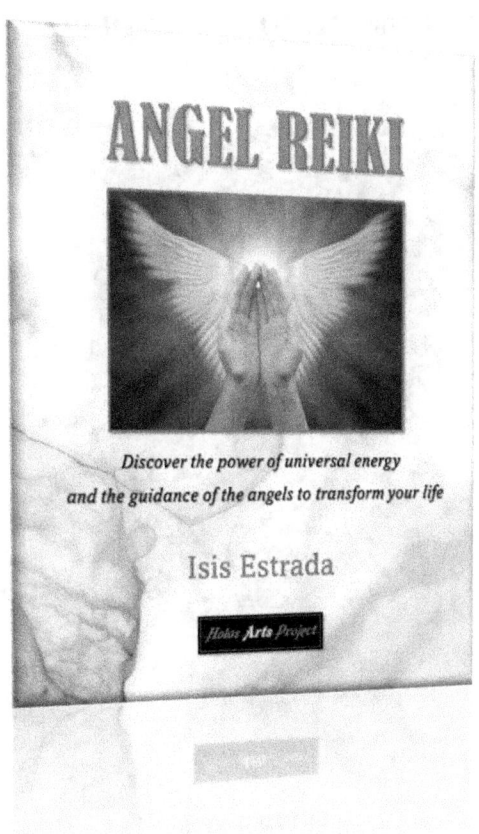

Angel Reiki

If you are looking for a new approach to Reiki that incorporates the wisdom and power of the Angels, you need to read "Angel Reiki" by Isis Estrada. This book will teach you how to connect with the Angels and Archangels and use their assistance along with Reiki energy to heal yourself and others.

RECOMMENDED READINGS

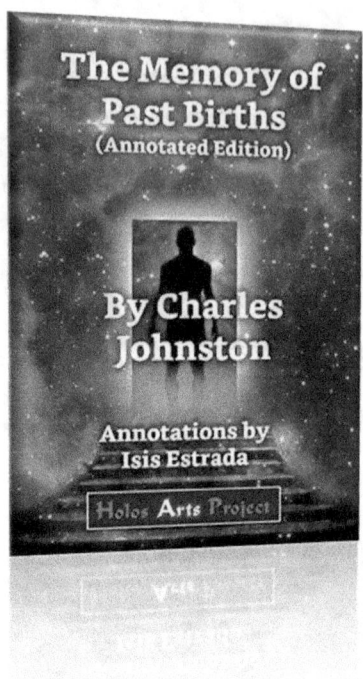

The Memory of Past Births, by Charles Johnston

Do past lives exist? And more importantly: How to remember them? Charles Johnston knew how to bring the millenary knowledge acquired during his travels in the East, and present it in his own time with much accuracy and certainty. Now, it is up to us not to allow his work to be lost, especially when it carries within its letters an inexhaustible source of wisdom for which we are still thirsty. We present, then, the first Spanish translation of *The Memory of Past Births,* which we are sure will become part of your favorite readings on the subject of transmigration, or reincarnation of the soul.

Buy it on Amazon, in print or digital versions.

https://www.amazon.com/dp/B0841FHB28

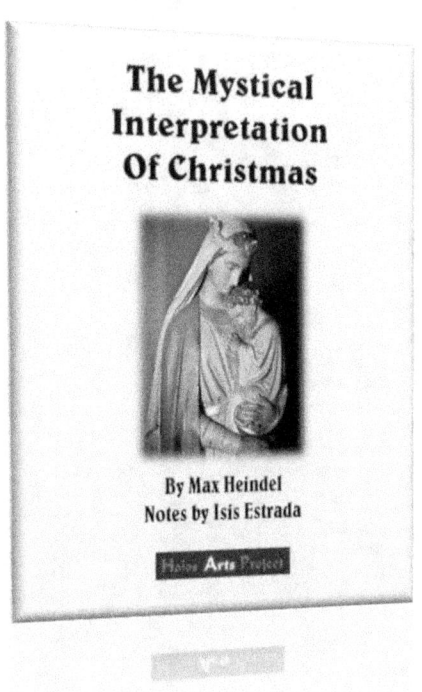

The Mystical Interpretation of Christmas

Of all the seasons of the year, Christmas season is the one that most rejoices our spirit and predisposes our soul towards the most beautiful virtues. A sense of hope and renewal fills the hearts, and an atmosphere of ethereal happiness permeates our homes.

Max Heindel, a notable Danish-American mystic, and member of Freemasonry and the Rosicrucian fraternity of his time, presents us with a text that elucidates the spiritual symbolism of Christmas, so as not to forget its deepest aspect in our lives.
Buy it on Amazon, in print or digital versions.

https://www.amazon.com/dp/B08P21GT9L

www.ingramcontent.com/pod-product-compliance
Lightning Source LLC
Chambersburg PA
CBHW062344290526
45794CB00005B/2102